Endocrinology

Case Studies in Reproductive Endocrinology

Shahla Nader MD

Professor of Obstetrics and Gynecology and Internal Medicine, University of Texas Medical School, Houston Health Science Center, Houston, Texas, USA

A member of the Hodder Headline Group
LONDON
Co-published in the USA by
Oxford University Press Inc., New York

First published in Great Britain in 2000 by
Arnold, a member of the Hodder Headline Group,
338 Euston Road, London NW1 3BH

http://www.arnoldpublishers.com

Co-published in the United States of America by
Oxford University Press Inc.,
198 Madison Avenue, New York, NY10016
Oxford is a registered trademark of Oxford University Press

Whilst the advice and information in this book are believed to be true and accurate at the
date of going to press, neither the author nor the publisher can accept any legal responsi-
bility or liability for any errors or omissions that may be made. In particular (but without
limiting the generality of the preceding disclaimer) every effort has been made to check
drug dosages; however, it is still possible that errors have been missed. Furthermore, dosage
schedules are constantly being revised and new side-effects recognized. For these reasons
the reader is strongly urged to consult the drug companies' printed instructions before
administering any of the drugs recommended in this book.

British Library Cataloguing in Publication Data
A catalogue record for this book is available from the British Library

Library of Congress Cataloging-in-Publication Data
A catalog record for this book is available from the Library of Congress

ISBN 0 340 75963 1 (pb)

1 2 3 4 5 6 7 8 9 10

Commissioning Editor: Joanna Koster
Production Editor: Wendy Rooke
Production Controller: Priya Gohil
Cover design: Terry Griffiths

Typeset in 11/13 Goudy by Saxon Graphics Ltd, Derby
Printed and bound in Great Britain by J.W. Arrowsmith, Bristol

What do you think about this book? Or any other Arnold title?
Please send your comments to feedback.arnold@hodder.co.uk

Dedication

This book is dedicated to the memory of my father

Contents

Preface

Gynecologists, endocrinologists and primary care physicians encounter many patients, particularly women, with reproductive disorders. The pathophysiology of these disorders encompasses both gynecology and specialized areas of endocrinology. As a result, many physicians are uncomfortable dealing with these patients and unfamiliar with their problems. This book is intended for such physicians. Discussions centered around case studies work through the different hormonal problems and common symptoms. Although some cases are not presented in great detail, they are none the less included because they provide grounds for discussion of important facets of reproductive disorders. The normal ranges of the most commonly used tests are listed in a separate table in conventional and SI units, and any departures from this range are indicated in the text.

Hypothalamic disorders

1

Case 1

An 18-year-old Asian woman attended because of primary amenorrhea. She was the product of a normal pregnancy. Childhood development was somewhat delayed but otherwise normal. She attended school at the age of 7 years and remained a good average student. There had been no development of pubic and axillary hair and no breast development, and she was still growing in height. Her past medical history was unremarkable, and she was on no medications. An injection of progesterone given 4 weeks prior to her visit had failed to induce menses. There was no family history of delayed menarche or other endocrine disorders; two younger sisters had already established menses at 12 and 13 years of age, respectively. She gave no history of galactorrhea, headaches, weight loss or excessive exercise, and her vision was normal, as was her sense of smell.

On examination, her weight was found to be 120 lb (54.5 kg), her height was 5 feet 6 inches (168 cm) and her blood pressure 130/85 mmHg. She had no skeletal abnormalities. Her span was 5 feet 9½ inches (176 cm). Her lower segment was 36½ inches (93 cm) and her upper segment was 29½ inches (75 cm). Her visual fields and fundi were normal. She had no axillary or pubic hair and no breast development, and her cervix and uterus could not be visualized or felt on pelvic examination.

Laboratory Tests

Luteinizing hormone (LH) was undetectable, follicle-stimulating hormone (FSH) was 0.8 IU/L, prolactin was 4 ng/mL, thyroid function tests were normal and testosterone was 5 ng/dL. Magnetic resonance imaging (MRI) of the hypothalamus/pituitary did not reveal any abnormality. Transabdominal pelvic ultrasound examination was unable to delineate a cervix or uterus.

Case 2

A 28-year-old Asian woman was seen because of primary amenorrhea and primary infertility. She was the product of a normal pregnancy and her childhood development had been normal. She had developed pubic and axillary hair in her late teens, but there had been virtually no breast development and no menses. At the age of 22 years, estrogen/progestin treatment induced her first menses and she continued this treatment until 1 year prior to her visit, with no spontaneous menses during this time. Her general health was good, and there was no history of galactorrhea or other reproductive symptoms. The only additional history was that of a significantly impaired sense of smell.

On examination, she weighed 113½ lb (51.6 kg) with a height of 5 feet 3 inches (160 cm). Her breasts were moderately well developed. General physical examination and pelvic examination revealed no abnormalities except for the inability to smell.

Laboratory Tests
LH was 1.2 and repeat 0.6 IU/L, FSH was 1 IU/L, prolactin was 15 ng/mL and estradiol was 2 pg/mL. MRI of the hypothalamus and pituitary was normal, and thyroid function was also normal.

Case 3

A 23-year-old patient was referred because of primary amenorrhea. She was the product of a normal pregnancy. Pubic and axillary hair had developed in her early teens. She also showed some breast development at this time. At the age of 16 years, progestin challenge failed to induce menses but she had a period on a cycle of estrogen/progestin. She had received no further treatment until a few weeks prior to her visit, at which time oral contraceptives have been prescribed for her. At the age of 22 years, an ovarian biopsy had revealed the presence of oocytes beneath the cortical surface. She was working as a physical education coach. There was no history of galactorrhea or weight loss. Her exercise history was as follows. Between the ages of 11 and 18 years, she engaged in 1.5 hours of volleyball, track and basketball per day. Between the ages of 18 and 21 years, she was running 5 miles (8 km) per week (although not on a regular basis), and at the age of 22 years, she stopped exercising for 2.5 months while recovering from surgery on her toe (for removal of a neuroma). At the time of her visit, she was on her second cycle of oral contraceptives.

On examination, she weighed 154 lb (70 kg) and her height was 5 feet 8 inches (173 cm). She had normal pubic and axillary hair and normal breasts except for small inverted nipples. General physical and pelvic examinations were normal, as was her sense of smell.

Laboratory Tests
Her oral contraceptives were discontinued. Her LH was 1.0 IU/L, increasing to 13.8 IU/L in response to 100 µg gonadotropin-releasing hormone (GNRH), her FSH was 1.3 IU/L rising to 4.9 IU/L in response to GNRH, prolactin was 5.3 ng/mL, estradiol was 15 pg/mL, and thyroid function tests were normal. She failed to ovulate or have menses in response to clomiphene, 100 mg daily for 5 days. An MRI of the hypothalamus and pituitary did not reveal any abnormalities.

Follow-up
She was treated with cyclic estrogen/progestin and had regular menses on this treatment. At the age of 26 years, she was taken off treatment for 2 months but failed to have a period. She was not engaged in any physical activity at the time.

FUNCTIONAL HYPOTHALAMIC AMENORRHEA

Case 4

A 17-year-old patient was referred because of secondary amenorrhea of 21 months' duration. Secondary sexual characteristics developed at the age of 13 years, followed by menarche at the age of 14 years. Although initially irregular, her menses were occurring monthly by the age of 15 years, and continued so for a few months until she became amenorrheic. Prior to the onset of amenorrhea, she weighed 120 lb (54.5 kg), was unhappy with her weight and started a diet, with a resultant weight loss of 50 lb (22.7 kg) during the subsequent months. There was no history of excessive exercise. However, there was a history of family conflict. At the time of her visit, she was unable to keep food down and would vomit after eating, this sometimes being induced in order to relieve fullness.

On examination, she was found to be emaciated and weighed 70 lb (31.8 kg) with a height of 5 feet 4 inches (162.5 cm). Her blood pressure was 88/48 mmHg, she had lanugo hair across her back and somewhat atrophic breasts without galactorrhea. Pelvic examination revealed a small uterus and no adnexal enlargement.

Laboratory Tests

Normal chemistry was found with normal T_4, T_3 resin uptake and TSH, but a suppressed T_3 of 0.75 ng/mL (normal range 0.9–2.0 ng/mL). Her baseline cortisol level was 13.6 μg/dL, increasing to 38.7 μg/dL in response to Cortrosyn stimulation. Her LH was < 0.5 IU/L, FSH was 4.1 IU/L, prolactin was 4.4 ng/mL and estradiol was 39 pg/mL. Computerized tomography (CT) of her brain revealed no abnormality.

Case 5

A 24-year-old patient was seen because of a 2-year history of amenorrhea/oligomenorrhea. Her menarche was at age 13 years, and she had 28-day cycles until the age of 22 years, after which she became essentially amenorrheic with only two menses in the preceding 12 months. There was no significant past medical history, but there was a history of an intensive exercise program over the last 2 years, which involved up to 3 hours of running and aerobics per day. There had been no significant weight change.

On examination, she weighed 135 lb (61.4 kg) and her height was 5 feet 8 inches (173 cm). She was clinically euthyroid with a palpable thyroid. Breast examination did not reveal any galactorrhea, and general physical and pelvic examinations did not reveal any abnormalities.

Laboratory Tests
Thyroid function tests were normal, prolactin was 8.1 ng/mL, LH was 3.5 IU/L and FSH was 4.0 IU/L.

Case 6

An 18-year-old patient was referred because of secondary amenorrhea. She was the product of a normal pregnancy but had developed infantile spasms at 5 months of age and was subsequently mentally retarded. She exhibited nervous uncontrollable behaviour. Adrenarche occurred at the age of 15 years, followed by some breast development. Her menarche occurred at age 17½ years and she had a second period 2 months later, this being followed by amenorrhea. There was no history of excessive exercise, but she had lost some weight since her mid-teens.

Examination
She weighed 91 lb (41.4 kg) and her height was 5 feet 1 inch (155 cm). She was euthyroid and had no goiter. Her breasts were developed but small with prominent areolae (Tanner stage 3). She had normal pubic and axillary hair, and a limited pelvic examination revealed a small uterus.

Laboratory Test
LH was 1.5 IU/L, FSH was 1.7 IU/L, estradiol was 10.2 pg/mL, and prolactin was 3.3 ng/mL, and thyroid function tests were normal. A gonadotropin-releasing hormone test of gonadotropin reserve was performed using 100 μg GNRH (Table 1.1).

Follow-up
She was initially given estrogen/progestin therapy. Her breasts developed further and her weight increased to 113 lb (51.4 kg). Her hormone replacement therapy was discontinued and spontaneous 28- to 32-day cycles ensued.

Table 1.1 Gonadotropin-releasing hormone test

Time	LH (IU/L)	FSH (IU/L)
Baseline	1.6	3.0
30 minutes	18.1	11.8
60 minutes	14.7	13.8
90 minutes	10.7	12.6

Case 7

A 27-year-old patient presented with an 8-month history of amenorrhea. Her menarche occurred at age 11 years. Her cycles were initially regular and painful, but by the age of 17 years she had become amenorrheic. She remained so until the age of 21 years, when birth-control pill therapy was initiated. She took this medication until 8 months prior to her visit, and she had no further menses. Two courses of medroxyprogesterone acetate failed to induce menses. There was no history of hirsutism, acne, galactorrhea or hot flashes. However, she gave a history of extensive exercise as follows. From the age of 16 to 27 years she was running up to 30–40 miles (48–64 km) per week. Twenty months prior to her visit, a car accident resulted in slowing of her physical activity and she was considerably less active at the time of her visit, but had lost 10 lb (4.5 kg), reaching a minimum weight of approximately 102 lb (46 kg). There was no history of an eating disorder, but she was on a strict low-fat diet.

Examination
She was thin, weighing 110 lb (50 kg), and was clinically euthyroid and had no goiter. There was no galactorrhea, and general and pelvic examinations were normal.

Laboratory Tests
Tests performed prior to her visit were as follows. Her LH was 3.7 IU/L, FSH was 4.7 IU/L, prolactin was 5 ng/mL, thyroid function tests were normal, estradiol was 19 pg/mL, testosterone was 16 ng/dL, dehydroepiandrosterone sulfate (DHEA-S) was 200 µg/dL, and the cortisol response to adrenocorticotropic hormone (ACTH) challenge was entirely normal. The only additional test performed was of bone mineral density, which showed a bone density of 79–84% of peak bone mass over her lumbar spine (at slight fracture risk) and 80–85% over her left hip.

Follow-up
Repeat medroxyprogesterone challenge was followed by menses, and one cycle of clomiphene stimulation using 50 mg per day resulted in ovulation and pregnancy.

Case 8

A 22-year-old patient was referred because of amenorrhea. Her menarche occurred at the age of 14 years, and she had regular 28-day cycles until the age of 18 years. At this time, her menses became infrequent and finally stopped at the age of 19 years. At age 21 years, she was hospitalized because of anorexia nervosa, and she received hyperalimentation. There was also a history of self-induced vomiting and laxative and diuretic abuse. Her lowest weight during the last 3 years had been 105 lb (47.7 kg). During this time she had also been running up to 20 miles (32 km) per week. Numerous cycles of medroxyprogesterone acetate had failed to induce menses.

Examination
Her weight was 124 lb (54.5 kg) and her height was 5 feet 7 inches (170 cm). Her blood pressure was 110/70 mmHg. She was clinically euthyroid and had no goiter. General physical examination did not reveal any abnormalities. A previous pelvic examination had been normal.

Laboratory Tests
TSH was 1.7 µIU/mL, LH was 5 IU/L, FSH was 4.3 IU/L, prolactin was 5.2 ng/mL and estradiol was 62 pg/mL.

Case 9

A 20-year-old patient was referred for evaluation of irregular menses. At the age of 12 years she had been diagnosed with juvenile astrocytoma that was affecting her cerebellum. The tumor was surgically removed and a ventricular shunt was placed. At the time of her surgery, she weighed 49 lb (22.3 kg) and slowly gained weight, so that she weighed approximately 100 lb (45.5 kg) by the age of 18 years. It was at this time that she had her first period. Since that time, her periods had been sporadic, occurring every 6–7 weeks. She had continued to gain weight and she ran 6–7 miles (10–11 km) per week.

Examination
She weighed 117 lb (53 kg) and was clinically euthyroid. General physical and pelvic examinations were normal.

Laboratory Tests
Thyroid function was normal, prolactin was 3.9 ng/mL and FSH was 3.4 IU/L.

Case 10

A 15-year-old patient was referred because of irregular menses. Her menarche occurred at age 9 years, and her menstrual cycles were irregular, with intervals ranging from 2½ to 5½ weeks. She had no galactorrhea, hirsutism or other symptoms. There was no history of weight loss, but she had been intensely involved in gymnastics, dancing and cheerleading in 6th to 9th grades (age 12–15 years).

Examination
She weighed 126 lb (57.3 kg) and her height was 5 feet 2½ inches (159 cm). She had Tanner stage III breasts and was clinically euthyroid. There was no excess hair, and pelvic examination was normal.

Laboratory Tests
Her thyroid function tests were normal. Her prolactin was 5.5 ng/mL, LH was 3.0 IU/L, FSH was 2.7 IU/L, testosterone was 6 ng/dL and DHEA-S was 167 µg/dL.

Follow-up
Over the subsequent year or so, she reduced her dancing, gymnastics and other physical activities and established regular menstrual cycles.

Case 11

A 33-year-old woman attended complaining of secondary amenorrhea. Menarche had occurred at the age of 13 years, followed by monthly periods. She continued with regular menses until the age of 31 years. In the 2 years preceding her visit she had only had three spontaneous menses. Her past medical history was significant for concussion at the age of 26 years and a weight loss of 15–20 lb (7–9 kg) over the preceding 2–3 years. She informed us that her present body fat was 19%. Her job involved physical education, and she had been engaged in intensive sports for the last 2.5 years. This included 6–8 miles (10–13 km) of jogging per day and 5 hours of other activities, mainly aerobics.

On examination, she weighed 140 lb (63.6 kg) with a height of 5 feet 8 inches (173 cm). Her breasts were somewhat atrophic and without galactorrhea, and she had mild excess hair. Pelvic examination was normal.

Laboratory Tests
Thyroid function was normal, prolactin was 5 ng/mL, testosterone was < 20 ng/dL, LH was 5 IU/L, FSH was 7 IU/L, and estradiol was 20 pg/mL. A lateral skull X-ray showed a sella turcica with a double floor. A CT scan was performed which showed that the sella was 60% empty.

TUMOR

Case 12

A 20-year-old patient was referred for management of hypopituitarism. Somnolence, vomiting and finally a seizure led to the diagnosis of a suprasellar germinoma. The patient underwent resection and this was followed by a dose of 5000 cGy to the primary tumor, 4000 cGy whole brain irradiation and 2000 cGy to her spine. Subsequent to this treatment, she received growth hormone for 2 years, her height increasing from 4 feet 11 inches (150 cm) to 5 feet 4 inches (162.5 cm). She also received monthly testosterone injections for a short time, to induce the development of pubic and axillary hair. She had no spontaneous menses and no breast development prior to her diagnosis. At the time of her visit, she was receiving hydrocortisone, thyroxine, cyclic estrogen/progestin and also desmopressin acetate. She had no visual deficit, but her right peripheral vision had been affected prior to surgery.

On examination, she was found to be clinically euthyroid and had no goiter. Her blood pressure was 125/80 mmHg. Her breasts were well developed and there was no galactorrhea. Her scalp hair was thinned, and her visual fields and fundi were normal.

Laboratory Tests
Serum sodium was 133 mEq/L, potassium was 4.5 mEq/L, creatinine was 0.7 mg/dL, serum osmolality was 279 mosm/kg (normal range 280–300 mosm/kg), urine osmolality was 950 mosm/kg, thyroxine was 12.8 µg/dL, T_3 resin uptake was 26%, free thyroxine index was 3.3 and cortisol was 2.8 µg/dL.

Discussion of Cases 1–12

During embryonic development, invagination of the ectoderm gives rise to the olfactory bulbs and tracts and to the arcuate nucleus that houses the gonadotropin-releasing hormone (GNRH) pulse generator. In this area, GNRH is produced, which is a decapeptide that binds to receptors located on pituitary gonadotropes and through calcium-mediated mechanisms affects the production, storage and release of the two gonadotropins, namely luteinizing hormone (LH) and follicle-stimulating hormone (FSH). Through central, inhibitory mechanisms and exquisite sensitivity to minimal steroidal feedback, the GNRH pulse generator is quiescent and inactive during the first decade of life. With the onset of puberty, these inhibitory influences decrease and the rhythmic pulsatility of GNRH becomes manifest, with approximately hourly release of small quantities of GNRH into the pituitary portal circulation. This vascular connection provides the necessary link between the arcuate nucleus and the gonadotropes. GNRH, produced in a pulsatile fashion, stimulates pituitary gonadotropin secretion (LH and FSH). Together these gonadotropins enable the growth and development of a dominant ovarian follicle, this being accompanied by an increase in estradiol production by the follicle. The mature follicle signals its readiness for ovulation by triggering a mid-cycle gonadotropin (particularly LH) surge, which enables rupture of the follicle, extrusion of the oocyte (into the fallopian tube) and formation of the corpus luteum. The corpus luteum produces progesterone which prepares and maintains the endometrium for implantation of the early embryo. In the absence of pregnancy, the life span of the corpus luteum is limited to approximately 2 weeks. Its hormonal production ceases, the endometrium is no longer supported and is shed, together with blood products, through the outflow tract. The hypo-thalamic–pituitary–ovarian axis is depicted in Figure 1.1 and the hormonal events of the menstrual cycle are summarized in Figure 1.2. Figure 1.3 is a schematic repre-sentation of the ovary showing the morphologic changes associated with folliculo-genesis, ovulation and corpus luteum formation.

Cases 1, 2 and 3 are all examples of deficiency of GNRH arising from an intrinsic defect known as primary hypothalamic amenorrhea. This disorder occurs with a frequency of 1 in 10 000 in men and 1 in 50 000 in women, and in men it is often called Kallman's syndrome. There are different modes of inheritance, namely autosomal dominant, autosomal recessive and X-linked recessive. In the latter, a defect in a gene (the KAL gene) encoding a protein involved in neuronal migration has been demonstrated, accounting for the anosmia that sometimes accompanies primary hypothalamic amenorrhea, as in Case 2. In fact, the finding of anosmia in a young female with primary amenorrhea or a young male with hypogonadism is virtually pathognomonic for this hypothalamic disorder. The MRI may also be abnormal in Kallman's syndrome, with hypoplasia of the olfactory bulbs and tracts. Although the molecular defect outlined above may provide a mechanism for some patients with this disorder, it does not explain all cases of

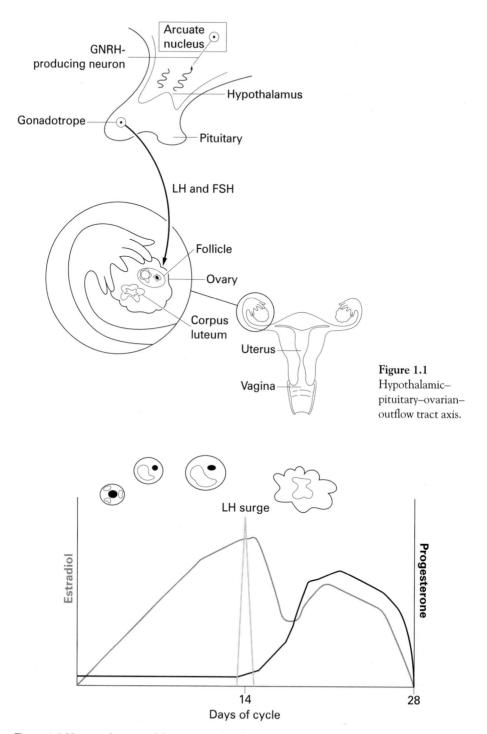

Figure 1.1 Hypothalamic–pituitary–ovarian–outflow tract axis.

Figure 1.2 Hormonal events of the menstrual cycle.

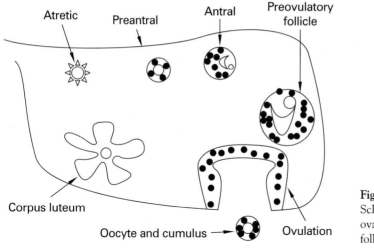

Figure 1.3
Schematic diagram of ovary depicting folliculogenesis.

primary hypothalamic amenorrhea. Patients with this disorder are often tall and eunuchoid in proportion (with the lower body segment more than 2 inches longer than the upper segment or the arm span more than 2 inches longer than the height) and virtually always sexually infantile with lack of breast development and small internal genitalia. This is well illustrated in Case 1, where the uterus and cervix could be neither palpated nor visualized on ultrasound examination, yet were clearly normal, as the patient readily established menses following estrogen/progestin treatment. Although the majority of patients are evidently hypogonad with lack of breast development, there is a degree of development in some, as in Case 3. This case is important because her low gonadotropins and primary amenorrhea with normal MRI (Figure 1.4) and prolactin and normal response to exogenous GNRH are highly suggestive of primary hypothalamic amenorrhea, yet she had a degree of spontaneous breast development and, in addition, a history of strenuous exercise that could also have led to amenorrhea, including delayed menarche. However, as her history evolved, it became clear that excess exercise was not the cause of her amenorrhea. In addition, she failed to respond to clomiphene challenge. While not all patients with functional hypo-thalamic amenorrhea (e.g. stress, weight loss and exercise) respond to the first course of clomiphene challenge, her lack of response was again consistent with primary hypothalamic amenorrhea, as clomiphene exerts its major effect on the hypothalamus, increasing the availability of GNRH. In patients with primary hypothalamic amenorrhea, ovulation can be induced by parenteral GNRH given in a pulsatile manner by means of an infusion pump.

In contrast, Case 4 is a clear example of functional hypothalamic amenorrhea. This teenager established normal monthly cycles but, concomitant with a history of very significant weight loss, she became amenorrheic. At the time of her visit she was amenorrheic, emaciated with atrophic breasts and internal genitalia, and had the lanugo hair typical of anorexia nervosa.

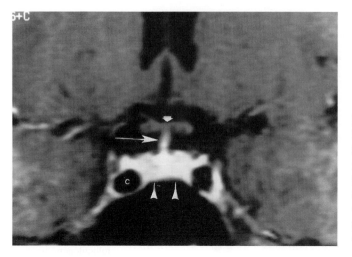

Figure 1.4
Magnetic resonance imaging (MRI) of a normal pituitary showing the optic chiasm (thick arrow), pituitary stalk (long arrow), pituitary gland (arrowheads) and carotid artery (C).

Case 5 is another example of functional hypothalamic amenorrhea, but this time related to excessive exercise. The timing of her oligo/amenorrhea coincided with her history of intensive exercise. Diminished activity of the GNRH pulse generator in this situation, like anorexia nervosa, appears to involve endogenous endorphins, corticotropin-releasing hormone (CRH) and possibly dopamine. Both endorphins and CRH are known to diminish GNRH activity. Weight loss, which often occurs in individuals who exercise strenuously, further exacerbates this situation, leading to more profound hypothalamic shutdown, as does stress. The three factors are additive.

Case 6 illustrates delayed puberty with very-late-onset menarche in a physically poorly developed and mentally retarded young girl. She, too, had low gonadotropins and an intact pituitary as evidenced by the very normal response to GNRH. After a few years of estrogen/progestin treatment, accompanied by significant weight gain, she established normal spontaneous menses, indicating that her original problem was functional hypothalamic impairment.

Case 7, which is again a clear example of functional hypothalamic amenorrhea, illustrates a few additional points. First, 30–40 miles (48–64 km) of running per week is certainly sufficient to shut down hypothalamic GNRH activity, and the time-course of the amenorrhea corresponded with the onset of her intensive exercise program. When she reduced her physical activity after her car accident, she lost 10 lb (4.5 kg) in weight, compounding her hypothalamic problem. Although she has no clear-cut eating disorder, she was obsessional about her food, severely restricting her fat intake and calorically keeping herself in a state of mild starvation. By the time she was seen, she was aware of some of these factors, had significantly reduced her exercise and, although her previous serum estradiol level was 19 pg/mL, which is extremely low, following her visit and some discussion she had progestin-induced withdrawal bleeding. This withdrawal was indicative of some degree of estrogenization of the endometrium – that is, some degree of recovery of her hypo-estrogenic state. The recovery is also manifest in her ovulatory response to her first course of clomiphene citrate, with ensuing pregnancy. In fact, her visit was prompted by a desire to become pregnant and her co-operation, in terms of increased caloric intake and reduction in exercise levels, was very strongly related to her intense desire to achieve pregnancy. She also illustrates a major problem linked to the hypo-estrogenic state of hypothalamic amenorrhea, namely reduced bone mass and bone loss. She had been amenorrheic for 4 years prior to treatment with birth control pills, and continued to be amenorrheic after cessation of this treatment. This duration of amenorrhea is quite sufficient to give rise to the increased bone resorption observed in hypo-estrogenic states.

Case 8 is an example of anorexia nervosa, bulimia and excessive exercise. Although bulimia is less often associated with amenorrhea than anorexia nervosa (presumably because bulimics generally maintain a higher body weight), it can be. In addition, this patient had been anorexic as well as bulimic.

Case 9 is an extreme example of delayed puberty and menarche relating to low body weight and lack of body fat. This patient only started menses after she had achieved a weight of 100 lb (45 kg) at the age of 18 years, and despite further weight gain, her hypothalamus had not fully recovered in that she was still oligomenor-rheic at the time of her visit. Her previous surgical treatment and her exercise regime may also have been contributing factors.

In Case 10, menarche occurred at the early age of 9 years. Although irregular menses and anovulation are common in the first year or so after menarche, this patient continued with irregular menses 6 years post menarche. Her dancing, gymnastics and cheerleading activities after her menarche appeared to be sufficient to decrease hypothalamic GNRH pulse generator activity, as evidenced by her recovery following reduction of these activities. Since in most adolescents these events correspond to the usual time of menarche (the age of approximately 12 years), delayed menarche is commonly observed in such individuals.

In Case 11, the history of weight loss and extremely intensive exercise is consistent with functional hypothalamic amenorrhea and a hypo-estrogenic state. However, radiologic studies led to the finding of an empty sella. An empty sella is not an infrequent incidental radiologic finding. The sella turcica may be empty (filled with cerebrospinal fluid) as a primary process due to a defect in the diaphragm sella, or as a secondary event, such as post-surgery, post irradiation, post infarction (Sheehan's syndrome) and following autoimmune lymphocytic inflammatory changes (e.g. in lymphocytic hypophysitis). The majority of patients with an empty sella do not manifest any endocrinopathies, but in a minority of cases, abnormal pituitary function (e.g. loss of gonadotropins leading to amenorrhea) is observed. Thus in Case 11, the differential diagnosis of functional hypothalamic amenorrhea vs. empty sella syndrome existed. The history of weight loss and, perhaps in particular, loss of body fat and excessive exercise coincided in time with the onset of this patient's menstrual disturbances, making hypothalamic dysfunction a more likely possibility. During the course of follow-up, this patient sustained a stress fracture and stopped exercising for a few

Box 1.1 Disorders associated with amenorrhea

1   Outflow tract and uterine target organ:
   - imperforate hymen – pain;
   - vaginal septum – pain;
   - müllerian agenesis – normal female phenotype;
   - testicular feminization syndrome – normal female phenotype but no pubic or axillary hair;
   - Asherman's syndrome – uterine scarring.

2   Ovary:
   (a) ovarian failure – absence of germ cells:
   - chromosomally competent: XX or rarely XY; primary or less commonly secondary amenorrhea, sexual immaturity with eunuchoid proportions;
   - chromosomally incompetent: XO Turner's or mosaic Turner's (XO/XX or rarely XO/XY), short stature, sexual immaturity and skeletal abnormalities;
   - premature ovarian failure (< 40 years):
     (i) infections (mumps, TB, possibly other viral);
     (ii) chemotherapy, irradiation;
     (iii) surgical;
     (iv) autoimmune disease (as part of polyglandular endocrine failure associated with primary hypothyroidism, Addison's disease, hypoparathyroidism, juvenile-onset diabetes mellitus;
     (v) genetic with family history.
   (b) ovarian unresponsiveness – inability to respond to gonadotropins despite presence of germ cells – rare;
   (c) disorder of folliculogenesis – chronic anovulation as in polycystic ovary syndrome.

3   Pituitary – lack of gonadotropins:
   - prolactinomas – micro- or macroadenomas;
   - hyperprolactinemia unrelated to tumor;
   - other pituitary tumors leading to hypopituitarism;
   - other space-occupying lesions – granulomas, metastatic tumors;
   - irradiation;
   - Sheehan's syndrome – pituitary necrosis postpartum;
   - lymphocytic hypophysitis – autoimmune inflammatory destruction.

4   Hypothalamus – lack of GNRH:
   - stress – functional amenorrhea;
   - anorexia nervosa or severe weight loss – functional amenorrhea;
   - exercise – functional amenorrhea;
   - space-occupying lesion – granulomas, meningioma, craniopharyngioma;
   - irradiation;
   - primary hypothalamic amenorrhea – Kallman's syndrome.

months. Her menses promptly resumed, confirming the functional nature of her reproductive disorder.

In Case 12, the absence of pubertal development, including adrenarche, thelarche and menarche was related to a structural defect, namely a suprasellar germinoma and its treatment (both surgery and radiotherapy). Post surgery, the patient was panhypopituitary and had diabetes insipidus. Her serum and urine osmolalities were indicative of adequate vasopression replacement using desmopressin. Her thyroid replacement seemed to be adequate, given her normal free thyroxine index (she was on estrogen, which increases binding proteins and leads to a high total thyroxine). TSH measurement is not useful, as this patient had secondary or tertiary hypothyroidism. An alternative method for evaluating thyroid replacement would be by measuring *free* thyroxine concentrations. Glucocorticoid replacement can be achieved with either hydrocortisone or prednisone. Prednisone is acceptable in this situation, as patients with secondary or tertiary hypoadrenalism continue to produce aldosterone because its secretion is not solely dependent on ACTH.

Box 1.1 outlines the causes of amenorrhea that are covered by these and subsequent cases.

2

Pituitary disorders

Case 13

A 37-year-old nulliparous patient was referred because of amenorrhea and an elevated serum prolactin level. Her menarche occurred at age 10 years, and she had irregular menses. These occurred every other month until the age of 14 years, at which time she became amenorrheic. She was evaluated at the age of 17 years. Although the details of this evaluation are not known, the question of pituitary disease was raised. She received one cycle of clomiphene and had two menstrual flows 1 month apart. Around the age of 32 years, she received three courses of Provera, none of which induced menses. She had no galactorrhea, headache or visual disturbances, and was taking no medications. Tests performed prior to her visit had revealed a prolactin level of 385 ng/mL, normal thyroid function tests, LH of 5.9 IU/L, FSH of 6 IU/L and an estradiol level of 52 pg/mL.

Examination
She was clinically euthyroid and had no goiter. There was no galactorrhea. Visual fields and fundi were found to be normal on clinical examination. Pelvic examination revealed a small uterus and no adnexal enlargement.

Laboratory Tests
Cortisol was 15.2 μg/dL. Repeat prolactin was 397.5 ng/mL. MRI revealed a lobulated 1.2-cm enhancing lesion in her right sella turcica, extending inferiorly into her sphenoid sinus and laterally into the cavernous sinus (Figure 2.1). A study of bone mineral density showed her to have a lumbar spine T-score of between −1 and −2.5.

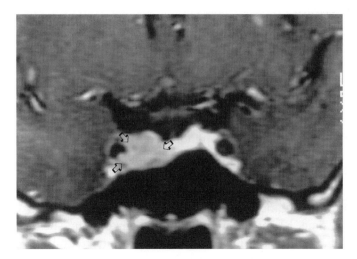

Figure 2.1
MRI of pituitary showing a
1.2-cm macro-
prolactinoma (arrows).

Case 14

A 33-year-old patient attended to seek advice regarding her amenorrhea and excess prolactin problem. Her menarche had occurred at the age of 14 years, and she had regular monthly cycles until the age of 20 years, when she started oral contraceptives. She took these until the age of 28 years, and was amenorrheic after discontinuing them. At the age of 29 years, she attended a physician, who found an elevated prolactin level of approximately 50 ng/mL. She was treated with bromocriptine after a plain X-ray had failed to reveal any enlargement or bony abnormality of the sella turcica. She became pregnant and had an uneventful pregnancy. She breast-fed for 3 months and was amenorrheic again until she desired a second pregnancy. At this time, her prolactin level was 104 ng/mL and she was given bromocriptine, resumed menses again and had a second uneventful pregnancy. She breast-fed for 6 weeks and was amenorrheic again until her visit to our clinic 2 years later. She had mild galactorrhea that was not troublesome to her, was not concerned about her amenorrhea and happy about her lack of need for alternative contraception. She was taking no medication, and the bromocriptine had been discontinued after the diagnosis of each of her pregnancies.

Examination
Her weight was 139 lb (63 kg) and her blood pressure was 100/70 mmHg. She was clinically euthyroid and had no goiter. There was readily expressible galactorrhea, and she was also moderately hirsute. Pelvic examination was normal and clinical examination of her visual fields and fundi did not reveal any abnormalities.

Laboratory Tests
Prolactin was 118 ng/mL, LH was <1 IU/L, FSH was 1.1 IU/L, testosterone was 43 ng/dL, and DHEA-S was 201 µg/dL. Thyroid function tests were normal. MRI examination revealed a 3-mm lesion in the right side of her pituitary fossa, consistent with a microadenoma (Figure 2.2). A bone mineral density study revealed densities consistent with her age.

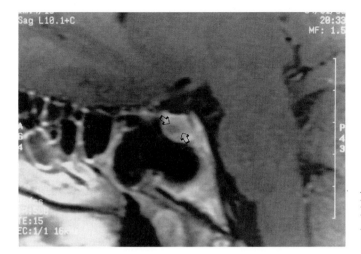

Figure 2.2
MRI of pituitary showing a
3-mm prolactinoma
(arrows).

Case 15

A 33-year-old patient was referred because of a 2-week history of headaches. She was 15.5 weeks pregnant and her reproductive history was as follows. Her menarche occurred at age 13 years, and she had regular cycles until the age of 30 years. At this time she became oligomenorrheic/amenorrheic and was found to be hyperprolactinemic (her prolactin level was 89 ng/mL). MRI revealed a 5-mm tumor with upward bulging of an enlarged pituitary gland, but no impingement on the optic chiasm. She was treated with bromocriptine, achieved normal cycles and subsequently became pregnant. The bromocriptine was discontinued at this time. Thirteen weeks into her pregnancy she had developed headaches and some nocturia. She had no visual symptoms.

Examination
The patient was clinically euthyroid. Her central fundi and visual fields were normal (confirmed by formal visual field studies) and there was no galactorrhea. Apart from enlargement of her uterus, the rest of her examination was unremarkable.

Laboratory Tests
Prolactin was 100 ng/mL, thyroid function tests were normal, cortisol was 12.3 μg/dL (afternoon cortisol) and her serum and urine osmolalities were 284 mosm/L (normal range 275–295 mosm/L) and 579 mosm/L (normal range 50–1400 mosm/L), respectively. MRI without gadolinium contrast revealed an intrasellar adenoma measuring 8 × 7 × 5 mm and displacing the normal pituitary superiorly.

Case 16

A 29-year-old was referred for management of her pituitary tumor. Her menarche occurred at the age of 12 years, and she had regular menses until the age of 16 years, when they became longer in intervals with occasional skipping. She was placed on oral contraceptives, and continued on them for 5 years. During this time, she developed galactorrhea which continued even after she came off the oral contraceptives. After stopping these pills, she remained amenorrheic. Investigations revealed a high prolactin level (approximately 80 ng/mL) and MRI showed a 5-mm pituitary tumor. She was treated with bromocriptine and established normal cycles and subsequently a pregnancy. Her pregnancy was uneventful and she breast-fed for 6 weeks.

Examination
Her visual fields and fundi were normal. She had bilateral galactorrhea.

Laboratory Tests
Her prolactin level 4 weeks after cessation of breast-feeding was 26 ng/mL.

Case 17

A 17-year-old patient was referred because of primary amenorrhea. In addition, she had noted galactorrhea for approximately 2 years. Her childhood development had been normal, breast development occurred at the age of 10 years and pubic and axillary hair development occurred shortly afterwards. There was no other significant past medical history, and she did not complain of headaches or visual disturbances. She was not on any medications. There was no history of weight loss, but she was fairly intensively involved in dancing and performing for several hours per day.

Examination
Her height was 5 feet 5 inches (165 cm) and her arm span was 5 feet 8.5 inches (174 cm). She was clinically euthyroid and had no goiter. Visual fields and fundi were normal. Development of secondary sexual characteristics was appropriate for her age, and she had minimal expressible galactorrhea.

Laboratory Tests
Thyroid function tests, including TSH, were normal. Gonadotropins were within the normal range. Her prolactin level was 100.7 ng/mL. MRI of her pituitary, using gadolinium contrast, revealed a 1-cm tumor extending inferiorly into the sphenoid sinus with no impingement on the optic chiasm (Figure 2.3). Formal visual field testing was also normal.

Follow-up
Following low-dose bromocriptine therapy, her prolactin level decreased. She established ovulatory menses and her tumor decreased in size.

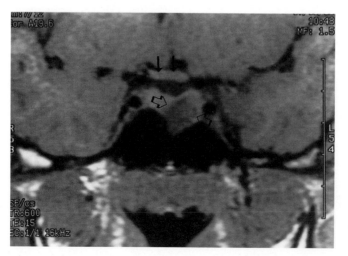

Figure 2.3
MRI of pituitary showing 1-cm prolactinoma (open arrows) and optic chiasm (closed arrows). The patient presented with primary amenorrhea.

Discussion of Cases 13–17

Prolactin is produced by the lactotroph cells of the anterior pituitary. Like all other anterior pituitary hormones, its production and release are governed by releasing and inhibitory hormones produced by hypothalamic nuclei. There are no direct neural connections between the hypothalamus and the pituitary, but there is a vascular link, namely the pituitary portal circulation. Hypothalamic hormones are released into the capillaries of the median eminence and the hormones are transported through a portal venous system into capillaries that supply the anterior pituitary. This important vascular link forms the pituitary stalk connecting the hypothalamus to the pituitary. The dominant hypothalamic control over anterior pituitary hormone production is a stimulatory one – that is, dissociation of the connection leads to a decrease in the anterior pituitary hormones LH, FSH, ACTH and related peptides, growth hormone and TSH. The only exception to this is prolactin, predominant control of which is inhibitory. This inhibitory hypothalamic hormone is dopamine. Thus severance of the hypothalamic pituitary connection leads to hyperprolactinemia.

Thyrotropin-releasing hormone – the hypothalamic hormone that controls TSH secretion – is also a prolactin-releasing hormone but plays a smaller role in normal prolactin physiology. In addition, lactotroph function is affected by the local hormonal environment. For example, hyperestrogenemia stimulates prolactin production and release by priming the lactotroph. This probably explains the 10-fold increase in prolactin levels during normal pregnancy. In a prepared breast (i.e. a breast exposed to some estrogen, cortisol, insulin, growth hormone and adequate substrate), galactorrhea can occur in the face of hyperprolactinemia. However, the absence of galactorrhea does not rule out an excess prolactin problem. Finally, hyperprolactinemia itself affects hypothalamic function by decreasing the pulsatile release of gonadotropin-releasing hormone (GNRH). Lack of GNRH is the most important mechanism leading to oligomenorrhea/amenorrhea or hypogonadism in such situations. Excess prolactin also directly inhibits gonadal steroidogenesis and may possibly have a local paracrine effect on the gonadotrophs. However, as indicated above, its most important inhibitory effect is on hypothalamic GNRH production.

Prolactin-producing tumors (prolactinomas) are a common cause of hyperprolactinemia, and indeed are the commonest pituitary tumors. They usually occur sporadically, but may be familial as part of multiple endocrine neoplasia, type I syndrome, together with hyperparathyroidism and pancreatic tumors. Prolactinomas may be less than 1 cm (microadenomas) or greater than 1 cm (macroadenomas) in diameter. Cases 13–17 all represent prolactinomas. Women with prolactinomas commonly present with amenorrhea (as in Cases 13–15) or may present with galactorrhea (as in Case 17, and also Case 16, who developed galactorrhea on oral contraceptives, but this continued despite cessation of the contraceptives). Occasionally, as in Case 17, prolactinomas may present with primary amenorrhea. Cases 14–16 all wished to achieve pregnancy. Patients with micro-adenomas may safely be treated with bromocriptine, a semi-synthetic dopamine agonist that lowers prolactin levels, restores gonadal function and also decreases the size of the tumor by shrinking the cytoplasm for as long as it is given. An alter-native, longer-acting dopamine agonist called cabergoline is also now available. It is especially suitable for patients who are intolerant of bromocriptine. Once preg-nancy is established, bromocriptine is discontinued. Although there is a small prob-ability of tumor expansion, presumably related to the hyperestrogenic state, this is uncommon, and it occurs in less than 5% of microadenoma cases. Patients are ques-tioned regarding symptoms of tumor expansion (namely headaches, polyuria and thirst from diabetes insipidus, and visual disturbances). Visual fields can be obtained at each trimester. When the patient becomes symptomatic, as in Case 15, prolactin levels can be measured and an MRI performed. Evidence of tumor expansion, using the above parameters, may necessitate intervention. Bromocriptine (or cabergoline) is the treatment of choice, not because of its prolactin-reducing effects but because it shrinks the tumor. If there are visual disturbances, a glucocorticoid such as dexamethasone may also be administered to help to reduce swelling and pressure on the optic pathways.

Trans-sphenoidal surgery is only performed in pregnancy if bromocriptine with or without glucocorticoids fails to resolve the patient's symptoms. Prolactinoma patients who have undergone a normal pregnancy can be allowed to breast-feed, as suckling does not appear to lead to any tumor enlargement. In addition, further pregnancies are not contraindicated in these patients. Details of the management of patients with prolactinomas who wish to achieve pregnancy are shown in Table 2.1.

Macroprolactinoma patients who wish to become pregnant present a different situation (Table 2.1). Although bromocriptine (or cabergoline) treatment will usually lead to restoration of gonadal function, because of their larger size there is a greater likelihood of tumor expansion (approximately 15–30%). As this is an unac-ceptably high rate of complications, the safest treatment in such patients is trans-sphenoidal hypophysectomy followed by bromocriptine treatment if needed (if cure

Table 2.1 Recommendations for treatment of patients with prolactinomas who desire pregnancy

Treatment	Microadenomas	Macroadenomas
Primary	Bromocriptine or cabergoline	Trans-sphenoidal surgery followed by bromocriptine or cabergoline (if necessary)
Alternative	Trans-sphenoidal surgery followed by bromocriptine (if necessary)	• Radiotherapy plus bromocriptine or cabergoline • Continuous bromocriptine (see text)

has not been achieved). In patients treated surgically as such, the tumor complication rate during pregnancy is less than 5%. In some countries the physician may opt to treat macroprolactinoma patients with continuous bromocriptine throughout pregnancy, to avoid tumor complications. Although bromocriptine is not mutagenic or embryotoxic and does not appear to cause congenital malformations, it does cross the placenta and its safety when given throughout pregnancy has not been established in large numbers of patients. For details of the management of patients with prolactinomas during pregnancy, see Table 2.2.

In patients who do not wish to become pregnant, amenorrhea is the rule. Although these patients are often happy to be amenorrheic, their amenorrhea represents a hypo-estrogenic state, with all of its attendant consequences, especially on bone. Although this situation can be alleviated by exogenous estrogen therapy, as estrogen may cause tumor growth this cannot be recommended as definitive therapy without some risk and very careful follow-up. Again, the alternative treatments are bromocriptine (or cabergoline) or trans-sphenoidal surgery. Both are acceptable for the management of micro- and macroprolactinomas, and dopamine agonists are usually the treatment of choice. In patients with significant visual disturbances, surgery is preferable. Macroprolactinomas that are operated on are often not cured, and even when they are cured, the patient faces a substantial recurrence rate. Microprolactinomas, especially those with serum prolactin concentrations less than 200 ng/mL, are more amenable to surgical cure. Radiotherapy, using either conventional external-beam cobalt therapy or concentrated irradiation with the gamma knife, may also be given either alone or adjunctively with surgery. Careful consideration needs to be given to dosimetry and safety when using the gamma knife, as some of these tumors lie quite close to the optic chiasm. Since bromocriptine leads to the re-establishment of menses, the hypo-estrogenic state is alleviated. In Case 13, the long duration of hypo-estrogenic

Table 2.2 Management of patients harboring prolactinomas during pregnancy

	Microadenomas	Macroadenomas
Asymptomatic patient	*Stop* bromocriptine/cabergoline Routine obstetric care with evaluation for symptoms of tumor expansion Check visual fields each trimester or if symptomatic	*Stop* bromocriptine/cabergoline Monthly evaluation for symptoms of tumor expansion Check visual fields each month
Symptomatic patient	Check visual fields Measure serum prolactin concentration Magnetic resonance imaging of pituitary gland Initiate bromocriptine with or without dexamethasone for visual complications Trans-sphenoidal surgery if unresponsive to bromocriptine	

amenorrhea almost certainly contributed to this patient's diminished bone density at the age of 37 years. She responded very well to 7.5 mg of bromocriptine, given in divided doses with food, and has re-established normal menses. Although clomiphene citrate may increase GNRH availability and lead to ovulation in some patients, as it did early in the course of this patient's disease, it is not the drug of choice and may not work when GNRH secretion is profoundly inhibited.

With long-term bromocriptine therapy, the dose can often be reduced over time and the same beneficial effect maintained. This 'improved' effect is almost certainly related to more permanent effects of bromocriptine. Long-term treatment may lead to fibrosis and, although this can be useful as the dose necessary to maintain euprolactinemia can be reduced, it can render any subsequent surgical treatment more difficult, and the surgeon needs to be aware of this.

In the evaluation and management of all pituitary tumors, consideration needs to be given not only to the possibility of a hormone excess state but also, because of the location of the tumor and a possible mass effect, to the effect of pressure on vital structures. Thus a tumor with suprasellar extension may cause bitemporal hemianopsia (because of compression of crossing fibers in the optic chiasm), or pressure may occur predominantly on one optic nerve. Lateral extension towards the cavernous sinus may lead to external ocular muscle palsies, and posterior expansion may affect the production of vasopressin, leading to diabetes insipidus. In addition, compression of normal pituitary by the tumor may lead to varying degrees of hypopituitarism. Pituitary reserve may be tested by evaluating the function of target organs such as gonads, adrenal glands and thyroid at baseline or a combined test of pituitary function may be performed as described in Case 29 on p. 49 and in the Glossary of Common Tests at the end of this book (p. 213). The majority of prolactinomas do not cause hypopituitarism, both because a significant amount of pituitary has to be destroyed for hormonal deficiency to be manifested and because the interruption of gonadal function by hyperprolactinemia usually leads to fairly early diagnosis. Hormonally functionless pituitary tumors, on the other hand, may grow to a larger size before manifesting themselves, and are more likely to be associated with visual disturbances and hypopituitarism. In patients who are hypopituitary, as well as restoration of gonadal hormones, glucocorticoids and thyroxine need to be replaced. A typical patient may receive 30 mg hydrocortisone in divided doses (or alternatively prednisone, 7.5 mg) and 100 μg L-thyroxine.

HYPERPROLACTINEMIA: OTHER CAUSES

Case 18

A 43-year-old was referred with a 1-year history of irregular menses and hot flashes. Her menarche occurred at age 11 and was followed by regular monthly menses until one year prior. At this time, she also complained of hot flashes. Laboratory tests had confirmed a menopausal status (FSH 44 IU/L) but had also shown a mildly elevated prolactin of 22.1 ng/mL (normal to 20 ng/mL), along with normal thyroid function tests. In view of this prolactin, an MRI had been done and had shown a 3 mm mass in the left superior aspect of the pituitary stalk. Her medications included carbamazepine and Tranxene. There had been a history of DES exposure in utero.

Examination
She was clinically euthyroid and had no goiter. Visual fields and fundi were normal. There was no galactorrhea. Pelvic exam revealed an upper vaginal ring but otherwise no abnormalities.

Laboratory Tests
A thyrotropin (TRH) stimulation test was performed; 500 µg TRH were injected at zero time. Baseline prolactin values were 14.8 and 11.9 ng/mL, with a peak prolactin response of 61.6 ng/mL at 30 minutes, returning to 30 ng/mL at 90 minutes. The MRI was reviewed by a neuroradiologist and the lesion was considered to represent a Rathke's cleft cyst.

Case 19

A 33-year-old was referred because of hyperprolactinemia. Her menarche occurred at age 11 years, and she had regular menses until the age of 16 years. At this time, her menses became irregular, heavy and prolonged, and over the years she required numerous courses of medroxyprogesterone acetate to induce menses. She had achieved pregnancy three times, but all of these resulted in miscarriages. Four months prior to her visit, she had noted galactorrhea, and a prolactin determination revealed a value of 63.2 ng/mL. She continued to be oligomenorrheic and in addition had had acne and hirsutism for most of her adult life. Her major past medical history was that of pseudotumor cerebri, diagnosed at the age of 26 years requiring eight spinal taps for treatment.

Examination
Her weight was 203 lb (92 kg) and her blood pressure was 120/80 mmHg. She had acanthosis nigricans and was moderately hirsute. Breast examination did not reveal galactorrhea, and a recent pelvic examination and pelvic ultrasound had been normal.

Laboratory Tests
Thyroid function tests were normal. Her testosterone level was 65 ng/dL, DHEA-S was 170 μg/dL, LH was 0.8 IU/L and FSH was 2.9 IU/L. A thyrotropin-releasing hormone (TRH) test of prolactin release was performed. After obtaining baseline samples, 500 μg TRH were injected intravenously and samples were obtained every 30 minutes for 90 minutes. Her baseline prolactin levels were 85 and 83 ng/mL, with a peak following TRH of 120 ng/mL, returning to 90 ng/mL at 90 minutes. MRI of her pituitary and suprasellar region was performed, which showed a mildly increased amount of cerebrospinal fluid within the sella, suggesting mild herniation of the diaphragm sella.

Case 20

A 28-year-old patient was referred because of a prolactin problem. Her menarche occurred at age 15 years, and she had irregular menses, settling to once every 30–60 days. At the age of 21 years, she took oral contraceptives for a few months but resumed her previous irregular cycles. At the age of 25 years, she noticed breast discharge, and had her prolactin levels measured, which were found to be high at 63 ng/mL. She was given bromocriptine for a while, which normalized her prolactin levels but not her menses. A computerized tomography scan performed in her local town had shown a sellar mass. She had occasional headaches, and had gained 40 lb (18 kg) since the age of 15 years. At the time of her visit, she had not been taking bromocriptine for 18 months.

Examination
She was overweight at 181 lb (82 kg) and was clinically euthyroid. She was moderately hirsute and had bilateral expressible galactorrhea. Visual fields and fundi were normal on clinical examination and pelvic examination did not reveal any abnormalities.

Laboratory Tests
Her thyroid function tests were normal, LH was 5.3 IU/L, FSH was 7.6 IU/L, DHEA-S was 284 µg/dL and testosterone was 83 ng/dL. A thyrotropin-releasing hormone (TRH) test of prolactin release was performed; 500 µg/dL TRH were injected intravenously and prolactin levels were determined at baseline and following TRH. Baseline prolactin levels were 39 and 37 ng/mL, with values of 67, 49 and 46 ng/mL at 20, 60 and 90 minutes post TRH, respectively. MRI showed a 13×10×10 mm lesion in the right side of her sella turcica, which was upwardly convex and causing stalk deviation.

Follow-up
Trans-sphenoidal surgery was performed and a Rathke's pouch cyst was removed. The patient's postoperative prolactin level was 1 ng/mL. Although her prolactin level remained normal, she was still oligomenorrheic.

Case 21

A 33-year-old patient was referred because of amenorrhea and galactorrhea of several months' duration. A prolactin level was obtained which was found to be considerably elevated at 213 ng/mL. She had had three pregnancies and continued to have regular menstrual cycles until a few months before her visit. There was a history of psychiatric disorder for which she was receiving treatment. This treatment was modified at about the same time as her history of galactorrhea, and included dopamine antagonists. At the time of her visit, she had been off her neuroleptics for 2 weeks. MRI studies had been performed which did not show any significant lesion.

Examination
The patient was clinically euthyroid and examination was normal apart from bilateral expressible galactorrhea.

Laboratory Tests
Thyroid function tests were normal. Repeat prolactin was 23 ng/mL.

Case 22

A 29-year-old patient was seen for hormonal evaluation during her second pregnancy at 35 weeks. After a normal menarche, she had regular menstrual cycles and achieved her first pregnancy at the age of 21 years. A year later a right temporal astrocytoma was found and partially resected. This was followed by 7 weeks of radiotherapy involving both sides of her brain. Within 18 months of her radiation treatment, she developed galactorrhea and her menses became sporadic. Her prolactin level was found to be elevated and MRI was performed. It was apparently abnormal and there was some debate as to whether the abnormality represented a pituitary adenoma or scar tissue. The patient was treated with bromocriptine, and although her prolactin normalized, her menses did not resume, and in fact she became amenorrheic. Meanwhile she gained weight and investigations performed locally revealed an underactive thyroid, so she was placed on thyroid medication. She was fatigued, and further testing revealed inadequate cortisol production and she was placed on hydrocortisone. Because she desired pregnancy, she had sought assistance. After clomiphene treatment failed to induce ovulation, she was treated with human menopausal gonadotropins and achieved her second pregnancy. She did not have visual disturbances or headaches.

Examination
Her weight was 195 lb (88.6 kg), and her blood pressure was 122/78 mmHg lying and 116/74 mmHg standing. She was clinically euthyroid and had no goiter. There was no galactorrhea, and her visual fields and fundi were normal.

Discussion of Cases 18–22

Apart from prolactinomas, there are numerous other causes of hyperpro-lactinemia. These are outlined in Box 2.1. The prolactin excess observed in these circumstances is self-evident, given the physiology of prolactin secretion and its control. There are numerous medications that may elevate prolactin levels, the most important of which are the dopamine antagonists, such as neuroleptics used in psychiatric disorders. This is illustrated by Case 21, where the patient had an extremely high prolactin level of 213 ng/mL, and was not surprisingly amenorrheic. Two weeks after coming off neuroleptics, her prolactin level was 23 ng/mL. Although prolactin concentrations in excess of 100 ng/mL raise the suspicion of a prolactinoma, this is not always the case, as illustrated here. Medications such as thorazine and haloperidol almost always increase serum prolactin levels, particularly during the initial phase of administration. Other medications used in psychiatry, such as antidepressants (including serotonin reuptake inhibitors) may also elevate prolactin levels, although not to nearly the degree induced by dopamine antagonists. The management of patients on neuroleptics is problematic. First, fairly large doses of bromocriptine may be required to lower serum prolactin levels to within the normal range. Secondly, these large doses may reduce the efficacy of the dopamine antagonists, and bromocriptine should probably not be administered without prior consultation with the psychiatrist managing the patient. None the less, the patient cannot be left hypo-estrogenic, and, ultimately one may need simply to replace estrogen (e.g. by using birth control pills). Other medications that elevate prolactin levels include metoclopramide, estrogen therapy (e.g. birth control pills) and, to a lesser degree, cimetidine.

Box 2.1 Causes of hyperprolactinemia

1 Prolactinomas – microadenomas $\leqslant$ 10 mm in diameter; macroadenomas > 10 mm in diameter
2 Medications – dopamine antagonists such as phenothiazines and related compounds, metoclopramide, antidepressants, estrogen
3 Stalk and suprasellar disturbances reducing dopamine availability – granulomas (e.g. sarcoid), tumors (e.g. meningiomas), trauma, irradiation, stalk disturbance in association with an empty sella
4 Primary hypothyroidism – TRH stimulation of prolactin (as well as TSH) release
5 Polycystic ovary syndrome presumed to relate to the hyperestrogenic state
6 Miscellaneous – stress, surgery, breast stimulation, chest wall injury or lesions such as herpes zoster, renal failure
7 Idiopathic

Since dopamine inhibits prolactin secretion, it is not surprising that disturbances of the pituitary stalk may lead to hyperprolactinemia. This is illustrated by Cases 18–20. In Case 18, a very mildly elevated prolactin level had led to an MRI which showed a Rathke's cleft cyst in the region of the stalk. Two further baseline prolactin values obtained in the context of a TRH stimulation test were normal, and as prolactin is a stress hormone, a single mildly elevated measurement needs to be repeated. However, there is a possibility that the stalk cyst may have led to reduced dopamine availability and thus mild hyperprolactinemia. Rathke's pouch represents the invagination of epithelium that gives rise to the anterior pituitary during embryologic development, and residual cystic remnants can occasionally be seen, found either incidentally or as above. As indicated earlier, TRH stimulates prolactin release and a TRH stimulation test can give information about prolactin dynamics. Generally, prolactinomas which are autonomously functioning do not respond to TRH, but give a flat response. Other causes of hyperprolactinemia show a significant response, and occasionally there is hyper-responsiveness to TRH (loosely defined as a peak prolactin level exceeding 60 ng/mL in a patient with normal or near normal baseline prolactin levels). This has been associated with ovulatory disturbances which may be amenable to treatment with bromocriptine.

Cases 19 and 20 are more complicated. Both patients had hyperprolactinemia that was responsive to TRH. Case 20 had a Rathke's pouch cyst which was causing stalk compression. Her prolactin level normalized following bromocriptine treatment and later surgery, but her menses did not do so because she also had evidence of polycystic ovary syndrome (irregular menses since menarche, excess weight, hirsutism and elevated testosterone levels). Case 19 also showed evidence of polycystic ovary syndrome (irregular menses since the age of 16 years, excess weight, hirsutism, acne, acanthosis nigricans consistent with insulin resistance, and elevated testosterone levels). Polycystic ovary syndrome itself, in approximately 20% of cases, may be associated with hyperprolactinemia (see discussion of Cases 24 and 25 on p. 42). Although the precise mechanism involved is not known, it may relate to the relative hyperestrogenic state of polycystic ovary syndrome. Case 19 is especially interesting because this patient had two potential causes for hyper-prolactinemia, namely polycystic ovary syndrome on the one hand and stalk distur-bance resulting from the mechanical effect of an empty sella on the stalk – that is, stalk traction – on the other. She had pseudotumor cerebri, with attendant raised intracranial pressure, and was also obese, and in this setting any defect in the diaphragm covering the sella could lead to leakage of CSF into the sella and hence an empty sella (for further discussion of this aspect, see Case 33 on p. 55). Hyperprolactinemia is occasionally a manifestation of an empty sella, the mech-anism being as described above.

Case 22 presents a real diagnostic challenge. This patient presented with galact-orrhea, irregular menses and an ill-defined abnormality on pituitary MRI, but although her prolactin levels normalized on bromocriptine, her menses did not, and in fact she became amenorrheic. In addition, over the course of the subsequent year or so she became hypopituitary, requiring glucocorticoid and thyroxine replacement. It is very uncommon for patients with prolactinomas to develop hypopituitarism, as these tumors have to be very large and destructive for this to occur. As bromocriptine did not induce menses, she was given clomiphene. However, this did not make her ovulate and was unlikely to do so, as an intact hypothalamus and pituitary are needed for clomiphene to be effective. She only ovulated and achieved pregnancy following gonadotropin treatment, this directly stimulating her ovaries. By far the most likely cause of her hyperprolactinemia and her hypopituitarism was the radiation she had received earlier. Both the hypothalamus and the pituitary are radiosensitive (the hypothalamus more so than the pituitary). Thus it is possible to lose dopamine inhibition of lactotroph function and have hyperprolactinemia, together with loss of the releasing hormones such as TRH (with consequent hypothyroidism) and corticotropin-releasing hormone (with consequent hypoadrenalism). This uncommon case beautifully illustrates these events. In time, this patient is likely to become panhypopituitary as a result of loss of *pituitary* function.

Case 23

A 24-year-old patient was referred because of oligomenorrhea, hyperprolactinemia and an abnormal MRI study of her pituitary. Her menarche occurred at the age of 14 years, and she had regular cycles. At the age of 17 years, she started oral contraceptives and took them for 1 year. Upon discontinuation of this medication, her menses became irregular with increasing intervals. She attended a physician who found hyperprolactinemia, and an MRI was performed which revealed a small microadenoma. She was treated with bromocriptine and a repeat MRI still showed a microadenoma about 4 mm in diameter. The two MRI studies were of differing qualities and so were not directly comparable. Her menses improved on bromocriptine treatment. Additional history consisted of a weight gain of 100 lb (45 kg) and a 1-year history of excess hair on the patient's face and chin.

Examination
She was clinically euthyroid and had no goiter. Her weight was 274 lb (124.5 kg). She was mildly hirsute and had acanthosis nigricans. Her pelvic examination was normal, as were her visual fields.

Laboratory tests
She had been off bromocriptine treatment for a few months when the following tests were performed. Her LH was 7.4 IU/L, FSH was 5.4 IU/L, DHEA-S was 180 μg/dL and testosterone was 48 ng/dL. A thyrotropin-releasing hormone (TRH) test of prolactin release was performed: 500 μg of TRH were administered intravenously and prolactin measurements were taken at baseline and following TRH. Her baseline prolactin levels were 67 and 68 ng/mL, increasing to 121, 91 and 85 ng/mL at 30, 60 and 90 minutes post TRH, respectively.

Case 24

A 23-year-old patient was referred because of galactorrhea and hyperprolactinemia. Her menarche occurred at age 10 years, followed by monthly cycles. She had a miscarriage at the age of 19 years, and a pregnancy termination at the age of 20 years. At age 22 years, she noticed galactorrhea, but she was on no medications that might have elevated prolactin levels this time. She continued with monthly menses. She was seen by a gynecologist who found a prolactin level of 53 ng/mL (normal range <25 μg/mL), and a normal TSH. MRI studies of the pituitary were performed and did not show any abnormalities. Additional history included a 30 lb (14 kg) weight gain.

Examination
The patient was clinically euthyroid. Breast examination revealed pinpoint galactorrhea bilaterally. She was mildly hirsute.

Laboratory Tests
LH was 2.5 IU/L, FSH was 3.0 IU/L and testosterone was 56 ng/dL. The patient was asked to rest, and two samples obtained for prolactin 15 minutes apart had values of 7.3 and 6 ng/mL, respectively.

Case 25

A 32-year-old patient was referred because of irregular menses. Her menarche occurred at age 12 years, and she had irregular periods 2–7 weeks apart. She continued with irregular menses unless she was on oral contraceptives. Additional history included substantial weight gain and a history of acne and oily skin and hair. Test results that accompanied her showed an elevated prolactin level of 36 ng/mL, normal thyroid function tests, normal DHEA-S and an elevated testosterone level of 62 ng/mL. She was not on any medications that could increase prolactin levels.

Examination
Her weight was 213 lb (97 kg). She was clinically euthyroid, and had acne but no galactorrhea or hirsutism. Pelvic examination was normal.

Laboratory Tests
Repeat prolactin measurement was 18 ng/mL (normal range <25 ng/mL).

Discussion of Cases 23–25

Case 25 is a clear example of polycystic ovary syndrome. She had a history of irregular menses dating from the menarche, excess weight, acne and oily skin, and elevated testosterone levels. A prolactin value of 36 ng/mL was found, and this mild degree of hyperprolactinemia is fairly typical of polycystic ovary syndrome. Prolactin concentrations may fluctuate, as in this case, as her repeat prolactin measurement was 18 ng/mL, which is in the upper range of normal. In the management of the menstrual irregularities of these patients, bromocriptine should be given, together with medications such as clomniphene citrate if pregnancy is desired. Case 24 is similar, but the signs of polycystic ovary syndrome were less obvious. This patient actually had regular menses and was only mildly hirsute. However, her testosterone levels were mildly elevated and repeat prolactin measurements revealed episodic hypersecretion of prolactin.

Case 23 represents a challenge in differential diagnosis. This patient presented in her late teens with irregular menses and was found to be hyperprolactinemic. MRI revealed a 4-mm microadenoma and a diagnosis of prolactinoma was made. However, certain aspects of her case are more consistent with polycystic ovary syndrome than with prolactinoma, namely her 100 lb (45 kg) weight gain, hirsutism, acanthosis nigricans, and mildly elevated testosterone levels. In addition, her good response to TRH was somewhat atypical of a prolactinoma. Thus, it was unclear whether she had hyperprolactinemia due to a prolactinoma or due to polycystic ovary syndrome. It is quite possible that the tumor seen on MRI represented a non-functioning small adenoma or incidentaloma – approximately 10% of individuals harbor such pituitary 'incidentalomas.'

Therapeutically, this patient would respond to bromocriptine regardless of the etiology, but surgical treatment should be avoided in such cases as it may not correct the hormonal disturbances. The adenoma can readily be kept under observation with MRI examinations.

Case 26

A 40-year-old patient attended to discuss her reproductive disorder and hyperprolactinemia. Her menarche occurred at the age of 13 years, and her menses were never regular. She was investigated at the age of 27 years and hyperprolactinemia was diagnosed. A computerized tomography scan did not reveal a pituitary tumor, and she was treated with bromocriptine. She established normal cycles and became pregnant. She did not resume her bromocriptine treatment after this pregnancy, and continued with oligomenorrhea/amenorrhea. Her past history was also significant for Graves' disease treated with radioactive iodine, this rendering her hypothyroid. She was on thyroxine.

Examination
The patient was clinically euthyroid and had no goiter. She was not hirsute, had no galactorrhea, and pelvic examination was normal. She had thyroid eye disease.

Laboratory Tests
Her prolactin level was 125 ng/mL. Thyroid function tests revealed a suppressed TSH, and her dose of thyroxine was reduced. MRI examination of her pituitary gland with and without gadolinium contrast did not reveal a pituitary tumor.

Discussion of Case 26 and summary of evaluation of hyperprolactinemia

It is evident from the preceding discussions that there are numerous causes of hyperprolactinemia apart from excess production by a tumor. It is important to search out medications that elevate prolactin levels, rule out primary hypothyroidism (with elevated TRH leading to prolactin excess) and look for signs of polycystic ovary syndrome. A history of head and neck irradiation (with a reduction in the production of hypothalamic hormones such as dopamine), or the finding of stalk abnormalities such as an empty sella or suprasellar cysts or other space-occupying lesions may explain the hyperprolactinemia. Prolactin is a stress hormone and can be elevated during stress, so the circumstances under which the sample is obtained need to be documented. In addition, chest wall injury or breast stimulation can lead to hyperprolactinemia through neural mechanisms. Despite all of these causes, it is not unusual to encounter a case of hyperprolactinemia with no obvious etiology despite thorough investigation. Such cases are labeled as 'idiopathic'. A few patients with idiopathic hyperprolactinemia (perhaps approximately 20%) go on to develop visible tumors, but in the majority of cases follow-up does not delineate any known cause. In Case 26, the patient had irregular menses all her life, and apart from hyperprolactinemia and treated hyperthyroidism she showed no evidence of other hormonal abnormalities. Her prolactin levels were very high and within the range seen in prolactinomas, but two radiologic studies approximately 13 years apart had failed to reveal a pituitary tumor. Her menstrual disturbances were easily corrected with bromocriptine, and she had an uneventful pregnancy. This patient fits the label of 'idiopathic hyperprolactinemia'; it is possible that she has a different set point for prolactin secretion or some degree of lactotrope hyperplasia. The correct management of her case entails the administration of bromocriptine or cabergoline in doses appropriate to reduce her prolactin levels to within the normal range and establish normal menses.

CUSHING'S SYNDROME

Case 27

A 26-year-old patient was referred for evaluation of hormonal problems. Following menarche at the age of 13 years, she had regular cycles until pregnancy at the age of 22 years. She gained 50 lb (22.5 kg) in relation to this pregnancy, became amenorrheic postpartum and continued to lactate. An elevated prolactin level (51 ng/mL) was documented, and she was treated with bromocriptine but did not resume menses without the addition of a progestin. One year prior to her visit, she was diagnosed with hypertension, had been hospitalized for depression and had developed hirsutism and bruising.

On examination, she was plethoric, had a buffalo hump, was centrally obese and weighed 198 lb (90 kg) with a blood pressure of 130/70 mmHg on treatment. She had fresh striae and proximal muscle weakness, and during the course of evaluation she developed fresh bruises. A recent pelvic examination had not revealed any abnormalities. She was euthyroid and had no goiter. She had marked acanthosis nigricans and was mildly hirsute. She had discontinued her bromocriptine a few months previously and did not manifest galactorrhea.

Laboratory Tests

LH was 6.5 IU/L, FSH was 4.2 IU/L, testosterone was 162.7 ng/dL, DHEA-S was 170 μg/dL, prolactin was 35.2 ng/mL, cortisol (p.m.) was 21.5 μg/dL, thyroid function tests were normal, sodium was 141 mEq/L, potassium was 3.7 mEq/L, glucose was 65 mg/dL and creatinine was 0.7 mg/dL. Her urinary free cortisol was 226 μg/24 hours (normal range 24–108 μg/24 hours). Dexamethasone 0.5 mg was administered every 6 hours for 2 days, resulting in a post-suppression cortisol level of 13.6 μg/dL. A recent chest X-ray had been normal. Other tests were performed and the results were as follows: repeat cortisol 22.9 μg/dL (p.m.) together with ACTH of 150 pg/mL (normal range up to 60 pg/mL), cortisol 16.8 μg/dL (a.m.) together with an ACTH of 110 pg/mL. A high-dose dexamethasone suppression test was then performed, with 2 mg given every 6 hours for 2 days. This resulted in a cortisol level of 3.5 μg/dL, and a 24-hour urinary free cortisol level of 17 μg/24 hours. MRI of the pituitary revealed a left intrasellar mass measuring 1.1 × 1.4 × 0.7 cm, deviating the stalk to the right. There was some extension of the mass into the cavernous sinus and also downward into the sphenoid sinus. There was no suprasellar extension.

Case 28

A 30-year-old patient presented with increased facial hair, acne of recent onset, a weight gain of 15 lb (7 kg) over the previous year, and facial swelling. She also carried the diagnosis of borderline diabetes based on a glucose tolerance test. Her menstrual cycles were regular.

Examination
Her blood pressure was 106/80 mmHg and her weight was 137 lb (62 kg). She had fullness of the cheeks and a small buffalo hump. Apart from facial hair, she had a normal hair distribution pattern. General physical examination was otherwise unremarkable, as was pelvic examination.

Laboratory Tests
Her thyroid function tests were normal. Her serum cortisol level was 21 μg/dL at 8 a.m., 23 mg/dL at 9 p.m. and 16 mg/dL at 3 p.m. Her 24-hour urinary free cortisol (UFC) was 620 μg (normal range < 100 μg). Following 0.5 mg dexamethasone administered orally every 6 hours for 2 days, her serum cortisol level was 19 μg/dL and her 24-hour UFC was 500 μg. After 2 days of 'high-dose' dexamethasone (2 mg every 6 hours), her serum cortisol was 3.5 μg/dL and her 24-hour UFC was 140 μg. Computerized tomography of the brain revealed slanting of the sellar floor to the left.

Discussion of Cases 27 and 28

Case 27 is a case of Cushing's disease that is somewhat atypical in its presentation. The signs and symptoms of Cushing's syndrome are outlined in Box 2.2. Although hirsutism, amenorrhea and weight gain are observed in patients with glucocorticoid excess (Cushing's syndrome), they are not specific features – that is, they are also observed in the much commoner disorder of polycystic ovary syndrome. The more important features of Cushing's syndrome include thinning of the skin, spontaneous bruising, proximal muscle weakness and (when looked for) osteoporosis. In addition, hypertension, psychiatric disorder and glucose intolerance are often observed. This patient's plethoric appearance, buffalo hump, striae, muscle weakness and bruising were all consistent with hypercortisolism.

Box 2.2 Signs and symptoms of Cushing's syndrome

*Thin skin**
*Spontaneous bruising**
*Muscle weakness**
*Osteoporosis**

Hirsutism
Menstrual irregularity
Acne
Hypertension
Central obesity
Plethoric facies
Buffalo hump
Moon face
Striae
Glucose intolerance
Psychosis

* These important signs/symptoms distinguish Cushing's syndrome from other common causes of menstrual irregularity, hyperandrogenism, obesity, etc.

Case 28 is also a patient with Cushing's syndrome, but this time with a more typical presentation. New-onset hirsutism and acne in a 30-year-old should raise suspicion of Cushing's syndrome, as the other much more common diagnosis of polycystic ovary syndrome usually has a much earlier age of onset. This patient's loss of diurnal cortisol rhythm, her high 24-hour urinary free cortisol level and her lack of suppression with low-dose dexamethasone (2 mg daily) were all consistent with the diagnosis of Cushing's syndrome. The very significant suppression of serum and urine cortisol with high-dose dexamethasone (8 mg) was highly suggestive of pituitary-dependent Cushing's syndrome. A tumor is not always demonstrated by computerized tomography or even MRI, but the latter is a more sensitive study.

To diagnose Cushing's syndrome, two types of tests are used (see Glossary of Common Tests on p. 213). In the first, urine is collected for 24 hours and urinary free cortisol is measured. With standard assays, an excretion rate exceeding approximately 100 μg/24 hours is indicative of hypercortisolism. In the second, 2 mg of dexamethasone are given daily in four divided doses and the suppressibility of serum cortisol is observed; within 48 hours serum cortisol should be suppressed to less than 5 μg/dL in subjects who do not have Cushing's syndrome. This patient had both an elevated 24-hour urinary free cortisol value and a non-suppressed serum cortisol value. To determine the etiology of Cushing's syndrome (pituitary dependent vs. adrenal vs. ectopic source of ACTH), further tests are performed. A high ACTH, as in these cases, rules out primary adrenal disease. To distinguish pituitary-dependent (the more common type) from ectopic ACTH sources, a high-dose dexamethasone suppression test was performed. Dexamethasone, 8 mg, was given daily in four divided doses and the suppressibility of cortisol was observed. Significant suppression of serum cortisol and 24-hour urinary free cortisol (preferably > 90%, as in Case 27) is consistent with pituitary-dependent Cushing's disease. Stimulation with ovine corticotropin-releasing hormone (CRH) will also distinguish pituitary from ectopic Cushing's, as there is a much greater ACTH response to CRH in Cushing's syndrome of pituitary origin. The intrasellar mass seen on MRI in Case 27 provided further confirmation of this diagnosis. It is likely that this patient also had polycystic ovary syndrome related to her insulin resistance, as evidenced by her acanthosis nigricans and her very high testosterone and normal DHEA-S levels (for further details see discussion of Cases 59, 60 and 65 on pp. 101 and 108). Mild to moderate hyperprolactinemia may also be seen in the context of polycystic ovary syndrome.

Trans-sphenoidal surgery with removal of the adenoma is the treatment of choice in patients with pituitary-dependent Cushing's syndrome. In patients who are not cured, radiation treatment is administered. Radiotherapy has a much slower course of action and may eventually lead to panhypopituitarism. In patients with adrenal sources of excess cortisol (i.e. adenoma or carcinoma), the primary treatment is surgical. Adrenal carcinomas are very aggressive tumors and often present at an advanced stage with a large abdominal mass and abdominal pain. Ectopic ACTH Cushing's syndrome may be seen in association with lung cancer, pancreatic tumors, etc.

SHEEHAN'S SYNDROME AND HYPOPITUITARISM

Case 29

A 31-year-old patient was referred for evaluation of a history of 11 months of secondary amenorrhea. Menarche occurred at the age of 16 years with subsequent monthly cycles. Her first pregnancy, which was uneventful, occurred at the age of 23 years. Her second pregnancy, at the age of 30 years, was a complicated one. In this pregnancy, the patient presented at 36.5 weeks' gestation with a 1-week history of nausea, vomiting, malaise and abdominal cramping and a 1-day history of vaginal bleeding. Her initial blood pressure was 166/86 mmHg, and she was observed to be jaundiced. A diagnosis of pre-eclampsia and abruptio placenta was made and the patient was delivered by caesarean section for fetal distress. There were no intra-operative complications. Her postpartum course was marked by the development of acute fatty liver, severe ascites, a pleural effusion and decreased hemoglobin levels. On postoperative day 3, she developed disseminated intravascular coagulation and was bleeding from her wound site. During the following 20 days, she required multiple surgery to drain subfascial hematomas and perform debridement. She experienced massive blood loss and at one point her blood pressure dropped to 56/25 mmHg. She required 20 units of packed red-blood-cell transfusions and 22 units of fresh-frozen plasma over the course of 3 weeks. She recovered from the above problems, but remained amenorrheic for the following 11 months. Associated symptoms included cold intolerance, fatigue and decreased stamina. She did not breast-feed, but she described breast engorgement which disappeared within 1 month.

Examination
Her weight was 122 lb (55.5 kg) and her blood pressure was 90/70 mmHg without postural fall. Her breasts were normal and without galactorrhea. She had almost no axillary hair, and pelvic examination revealed a tiny uterus.

Laboratory Tests
Baseline hormonal determinations revealed low-normal estradiol, cortisol and thyroid function, and therefore a combined test of pituitary function was performed as follows: 100 μg of gonadotropin-releasing hormone, 500 μg of thyrotropin-releasing hormone and 0.1 units/kg regular insulin were administered with samples obtained prior to and following the above medications. The results are shown in Table 2.3. In addition, MRI showed a partially empty sella with slight invagination of the optic chiasm anteriorly into the pituitary fossa (see Figure 2.4).

Table 2.3 Combined test of pituitary function

	Time (minutes)					
	0	15	30	60	90	120
Glucose (mg/dL)	66		62	40	49	60
TSH (μIU/mL)	1.1	1.7	2.7	2.3	1.8	
Prolactin (ng/mL)	10.8	17	25.2		15	
LH (IU/L)	0.9	1.2	3.1	3.4	3.6	
FSH (IU/L)	5.1	4.9	7.4	7.8	8.5	
Growth hormone (ng/mL)	<1		<1	<1	<1	
Cortisol (μg/dL)	5			3	7	9
Thyroxine (μg/dL)	7.3					
T$_3$ resin uptake (%)	22.6					
Free thyroxine index (FTI)	1.6					
Estradiol (pg/mL)	18					

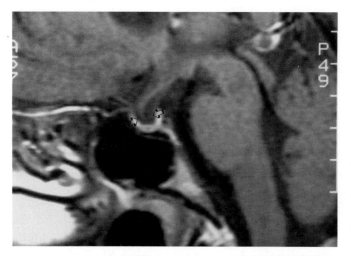

Figure 2.4
MRI of pituitary in a patient with Sheehan's syndrome, showing partially empty sella turcica (arrows).

Case 30

A 35-year-old patient was seen with secondary amenorrhea. She had been told that she had premature ovarian failure and she wished to conceive. Her menarche occurred at the age of 13 years and was heralded by a seizure. She continued to have seizures and required long-term medication for their control. She had regular menstrual cycles until the age of 27 years. At this time they became irregular, and by the age of 30 years she was amenorrheic and complaining of significant hot flashes. Although an elevated FSH level was never documented, she was diagnosed with premature ovarian failure and given estrogen/progestin replacement in cyclic fashion. Despite 0.9 mg of conjugated equine estrogen (CEE), she failed to experience withdrawal bleeding and her hot flashes were unresolved. Her past medical history was significant for a motor-vehicle accident, with head injury, at the age of 27 years. She had no neurological sequelae. Her past history was also significant for osteoporosis, presenting with backache at the age of 32 years. Despite her estrogen treatment as described above, she had continued to lose bone during the ensuing 3 years. At the time of her visit, her medications consisted of CEE 0.9 mg and medroxyprogesterone acetate (MPA) 10 mg, given in cyclic fashion. She was also taking 1500–2000 mg calcium supplements as well as phenytoin and phenobarbital.

Examination
She weighed 127 lb (57.7 kg) and her height was 5 feet 4 inches (162.5 cm). She was clinically euthyroid, had no galactorrhea and pelvic examination was normal.

Laboratory Tests
Her FSH was 0.5 IU/L, estradiol was 49 pg/mL, thyroid function tests were normal and prolactin was 3.4 ng/mL. Her CEE and MPA were discontinued for a few weeks, after which repeat FSH was 0.4 IU/L and LH was 0.6 IU/L. Her cortisol level was 16 µg/dL. MRI studies of the pituitary showed a very small amount of normal anterior pituitary tissue, and the signal pattern was consistent with previous hemorrhagic infarction of the anterior pituitary.

LYMPHOCYTIC HYPOPHYSITIS

Case 31

A 22-year-old patient was referred for evaluation of secondary amenorrhea and galactorrhea of 9 months' duration. Her menarche occurred at the age of 17 years, and she had normal monthly cycles. Her first pregnancy, which was uneventful, occurred at the age of 19 years, her second pregnancy at age 20 years was terminated and she had another uneventful pregnancy at 21 years of age. She did not breast-feed. A few weeks after delivery, she spotted for 2 weeks and then had no further menses. During those 9 post-partum months she had continued to lactate and had lost 29 lb (13 kg) in weight. Her past history was significant for sickle-cell trait and an episode of nausea, vomiting, fever and weakness 3 months prior to her evaluation. She had been hospitalized and treated with normal saline. Laboratory tests at the time had revealed a glucose level of 48 μg/dL, a thyroxine T_4 level of 1.7 μg/dL (normal range 4.5–12.5 μg/dL) and a normal TSH.

Examination
She was a thin, sick-looking woman with blood pressure of 104/62 mmHg. There was bilateral expressible galactorrhea. Pelvic examination was normal, as was examination of her visual fields and fundi.

Laboratory Tests
Her prolactin level was 60 ng/mL, and repeat measurement was 123 ng/mL. Her LH was 1.9 IU/L, FSH was 5.1 IU/L, cortisol was < 1 μg/dL, ACTH was < 25 pg/mL (normal range up to 70 pg/mL), T_4 was 3.3 μg/dL, T_3 resin uptake was 22%, free thyroxine index was 0.7 (normal range 1.1–4.4) and TSH was normal. Her serum electrolytes and glucose levels were normal. After injection of 500 μg of thyrotropin-releasing hormone intravenously, prolactin and TSH were measured. The patient achieved a peak prolactin concentration of 300 ng/mL and a delayed peak TSH of 42 μIU/mL. MRI examination of her pituitary showed an enlarged optic chiasm and thickened stalk which was retracted into a partially empty sella (Figure 2.5). Formal testing of her visual fields and acuity did not reveal any abnormalities.

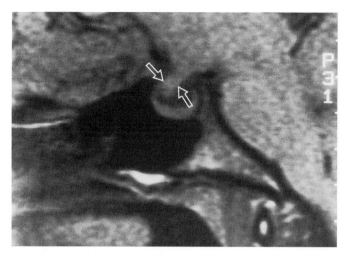

Figure 2.5
MRI of pituitary in a
patient with lymphocytic
hypophysitis showing
thickened pituitary stalk
(arrows) and partially
empty sella turcica.

Case 32

A 35-year-old patient was referred for hormonal evaluation. At the age of around 20 years she had been diagnosed with Hashimoto's thyroiditis and also immune-deficiency syndrome based on recurrent staphylococcal and fungal infections. Her menarche occurred at the age of 13 years and she had regular menses. At the age of 35 years, she developed galactorrhea and was found to have an elevated prolactin level of 80 ng/mL. At about the same time, secondary hypo-adrenalism was diagnosed and she was started on glucocorticoids. She was not taking any medication known to elevate prolactin levels. MRI had shown an enlarged pituitary with non-specific changes but no discrete mass. Her family history was significant for Graves' disease.

Examination
The patient was clinically euthyroid and had no goiter. There was no galactorrhea and her visual fields and fundi were normal. She had some moniliasis of her nails.

Laboratory Tests
A thyrotropin-releasing hormone (TRH) test of prolactin release was performed. After obtaining baseline samples, 500 μg of TRH were injected intravenously. Her baseline prolactin levels were 12 and 13.6 ng/mL with a peak prolactin value of 45 ng/mL at 20 minutes post TRH, and a value of 17.4 ng/mL at 90 minutes.

EMPTY SELLA SYNDROME

Case 33

A 33-year-old patient was referred for pituitary evaluation. Ten months previously she had had a molar tooth extracted, and had subsequently experienced intractable pain and consequently underwent numerous tests. These tests included an MRI examination which showed an enlarged and empty sella turcica. She had had regular menses since menarche, did not complain of galactorrhea and had no history suggestive of an endocrine disorder. She had two children, and the only obstetric/postpartum event of note had been pregnancy-induced hypertension. She remained hypertensive and was taking a calcium-channel blocker.

Examination
The patient was obese, weighing 255 lb (116 kg), and her blood pressure was 132/102 mmHg. She was clinically euthyroid and euadrenal. Breast examination was normal, as was examination of her visual fields and fundi.

Laboratory Tests
Electrolytes and glucose levels were normal, thyroid function tests were normal, cortisol was 15.7 μg/dL (noon), LH was 2.7 IU/L, FSH was 3.8 IU/L, prolactin was 5.5 ng/mL, and progesterone levels were indicative of ovulation. Her serum osmolality was 282 mosm/kg, and a random urine osmolality was 437 mosm/kg.

Discussion of Cases 29–33

Case 29 is that of a young woman with massive postpartum hemorrhage. Although her delivery was uncomplicated, within a few days she had massive bleeding that required multiple transfusions. She remained amenorrheic, and had cold intolerance and fatigue. Breast engorgement disappeared spontaneously within a few weeks. She had lost body hair and had atropic internal genitalia. A combined test of pituitary function was performed to evaluate pituitary reserve on the suspicion that she had hypopituitarism secondary to postpartum necrosis of the anterior pituitary (Sheehan's syndrome). Her baseline estradiol and morning cortisol levels were low and her free thyroxine index was low-normal. In response to GNRH there was a minimal rise in LH and FSH levels, and in response to hypoglycemia induced by insulin there was no growth-hormone response and only a minimal ACTH (and hence cortisol) response. In response to thyrotropin-releasing hormone (TRH) there was again only a minimal TSH response. However, the prolactin response to TRH was normal. Thus this patient had near total hypopituitarism and she was subsequently given replacement estrogen/progestin (in the form of an oral contraceptive), glucocorticoids and thyroxine. In such cases it is very important to replace glucocorticoids before replacing thyroid hormone, as thyroxine treatment alone can precipitate adrenocortical deficiency by increasing metabolic demands. This patient's MRI scan showed a partially empty sella, consistent with post-necrotic changes.

Sheehan's syndrome or postpartum hemorrhagic necrosis of the anterior pituitary is observed in 3.6% of cases of postpartum hemorrhage. Varying degrees of hypopituitarism ensue, as in this case. Clinically, they present with failure of lactation, postpartum amenorrhea and signs and symptoms of glucocorticoid and thyroxine deficiency. In about 50% of the cases, diagnosis is delayed for at least 10 years. In those who ovulate sporadically and achieve pregnancy, the pregnancy is complicated by the hypopituitary state, with a consequent risk of shock from adrenocortical insufficiency. The other major cause of hypopituitarism postpartum is lymphocytic hypophysitis. In such cases, a history of hemorrhage is absent. This is illustrated by Case 31, whose third uneventful pregnancy was followed by amenorrhea, galactorrhea and significant weight loss. She was also cortisol and thyroxine deficient. Her enlarged chiasm and pituitary stalk, which were retracted into a partially empty sella, were the most likely explanation for her hyperprolactinemia and galactorrhea, as stalk disturbances reduce the supply of dopamine, the prolactin-inhibitory factor. Her strong prolactin response to TRH was also consistent with a non-tumor cause of hyperprolactinemia. Her delayed but otherwise normal TSH response to TRH was also characteristic of a hypothalamic disturbance. Her nausea and vomiting were probably manifestations of cortisol deficiency. Fortunately, her low T_4 (found during hospitalization) was not treated with thyroxine. As she was also glucocorticoid deficient, treatment with thyroxine alone may have precipitated a crisis of adrenocortical insufficiency.

Case 30 is a complicated example of partial hypopituitarism manifesting as hypogonadism, and is presumed to have been related to the head injury sustained by the patient at the age of 27 years. The patient became oligomenorrheic and subsequently amenorrheic. Although her history of hot flashes at this time was highly suggestive of primary gonadal failure, her FSH level was never elevated – in fact it was always low. Primary gonadal failure cannot be diagnosed without an elevated FSH (usually > 30 IU/L), and since hot flashes are *hypothalamic* in origin, they can occur in the hypo-estrogenic state induced by hypopituitarism *in the presence of an intact hypothalamus,* as in this case. The MRI examination, which showed hemorrhagic infarction of the anterior pituitary, supported the biochemical findings of hypopituitarism. However, despite reasonable estrogen/progestin replacement, this patient failed to have menses, her hot flashes were unabated and she continued to experience bone loss. All of these were consistent with a continuing hypo-estrogenic state. In this context, it should be remembered that anti-seizure medications, particularly phenytoin (Dilantin) and phenobarbital, induce liver enzymes and thus increase estrogen metabolism. Thus the amount of estrogen being replaced was inadequate for her in view of her anti-seizure medication. When her dose of estrogen was significantly increased, she resumed menses, her hot flashes disappeared and her bone loss was interrupted.

Lymphocytic hypophysitis is a rare cause of hypopituitarism, with a predilection for women, often in the setting of pregnancy. It may present in the third trimester, with headaches, visual disturbances and hypopituitarism, masquerading as a pituitary tumor, or it may present postpartum as described in Case 31 with either hyperprolactinemia or hypopituitarism, or both. It is an autoimmune disease, and the finding of a personal or family history of other autoimmune diseases strengthens the diagnosis. Many patients with this diagnosis have ended up having pituitary surgery. A high index of suspicion for this diagnosis in a pregnant patient obviates the need for biopsy. Treatment involves the replacement of target organ hormones such as cortisol and thyroxine. Hyperprolactinemia will respond to bromocriptine and menses may be restored if their disturbance relates to the high prolactin level. Visual disturbances from an expanding inflammatory intrasellar mass may, in addition, respond to high-dose dexamethasone.

The patient in Case 32 has polyglandular autoimmune disease, which in some cases is associated with mucocutaneous candidiasis. She even has a family history of autoimmune disease. Her secondary or tertiary hypoadrenalism (that is, low ACTH and low cortisol) is suggestive of pituitary (secondary) or hypothalamic (tertiary) diseases. In addition, her hyperprolactinemia, as well as her enlarged pituitary without a finding of a discrete mass, were all consistent with lymphocytic hypophysitis, even though a pathologic diagnosis was not available. Indeed, her hyperprolactinemia resolved over time.

In Case 33, an empty sella turcica was incidentally discovered during the course of evaluation of a head and neck disorder. Empty sella syndrome is a fairly common disorder which is frequently brought to light incidentally as in this case. It is of heterogenous etiology. In the case of primary empty sella syndrome, a defect of the diaphragm sella (the membrane through which the stalk of the pituitary passes), especially when associated with hypertension and obesity, leads to the accumulation of cerebrospinal fluid (CSF) within the sella – hence the empty sella. The sella enlarges and the pituitary contents are pushed towards the floor of the sella. An empty sella may also be secondary to other causes, including surgical hypophysectomy, irradiation, necrosis (as in Sheehan's syndrome), or following inflammatory and autoimmune processes (as in lymphocytic hypophysitis). Pituitary function is usually entirely normal, as in this case, but occasionally varying degrees of hypopituitarism are seen (usually secondary hypogonadism). Occasionally the patients may have galactorrhea/hyperprolactinemia, presumably related to stalk disturbances and loss of dopamine (see discussion of Cases 19 and 20 on p. 37).

Ovarian disorders

3

CHROMOSOMALLY COMPETENT GONADAL FAILURE

Case 34

A 24-year-old patient was referred for work-up of primary amenorrhea. Pubic hair developed in her mid-teens, at which time she weighed 200 lb (91 kg). In view of her excess weight, assessment of whether breast development had occurred at this time was rendered difficult. At the age of 16 years, she attended a physician for primary amenorrhea. She was treated with continuous conjugated equine estrogens (CEE) for 6 months, followed by a few days of medroxyprogesterone acetate (MPA), and had a withdrawal bleed. Subsequently, she was placed on cyclic CEE, 0.625 mg, and MPA, 10 mg, and had monthly menses. At the age of 21 years, she discontinued her medications for 1 year without the occurrence of a spontaneous period. She then restarted her medications and continued them until she was seen at the age of 24 years. The only other past history of note was a 70-lb (32-kg) weight loss at the age of 18 years; she regained half of that weight over the following few months.

On examination, she weighed 174 lb (79 kg) and had a height of 6 feet 0 inches (183 cm); her upper segment was 33 inches (84 cm) and her lower segment was 39 inches (99 cm). She was euthyroid and euadrenal, and her breasts were well developed without galactorrhea. Her visual fields and fundi and sense of smell were all normal, as was pelvic examination.

Laboratory Tests
Thyroid function was normal, prolactin was < 3 ng/mL, LH was 71 IU/L, FSH was 66 IU/L, and lateral skull X-ray showed a normal sella turcica. Her karyotype was 46 XX.

Case 35

A 40-year-old patient with a history of primary amenorrhea was referred for hormonal management. At the age of 19 years she had presented to her physician with a history of primary amenorrhea and was found to have high gonadotropin levels. Her karyotype was 46 XX, and streak gonads were confirmed by ovarian biopsy. Hormonal therapy was initiated and she had received some form of estrogen treatment for approximately 18 of the 21 years that had elapsed since her diagnosis. Her estrogen dosage was inconstant and for the most part undocumented; she usually took very low doses to avoid breast tenderness and bloating. She always took a progestin. A bone mineral density (BMD) study 3 years prior to her visit had shown severe osteopenia, and a recent repeat study had shown no further change. The anterior lumbar spine and left hip BMD were both between –1 and –2.5 standard deviations below peak bone mass, that is, in the osteopenic range. She was a non-smoker, took 1 gram of calcium per day and reported a family history of osteoporosis. Her only other significant past medical history was that of ulcerative colitis necessitating eight courses of rectal steroids over the years.

Examination
Her weight was 131 lb (59.5 kg) and her blood pressure was 130/88 mmHg. She was clinically euthyroid and of normal height.

Laboratory Tests
Calcium, phosphorus, alkaline phosphatase and TSH levels were all normal.

Case 36

An 18-year-old patient was referred because of primary amenorrhea. Pubic and axillary hair had developed at the age of 12 years, and slight breast development had occurred at the age of 16 years. There was no history of chemotherapy, irradiation, galactorrhea or other major illnesses.

Examination
Her height was 5 feet 8 inches (173 cm). She was clinically euthyroid with normal axillary and pubic hair. Her breasts were approximately Tanner stage III, and she had no galactorrhea. General examination was normal and pelvic examination revealed a small uterus with no adnexal enlargement. Her sense of smell was normal.

Laboratory Tests
FSH was 74.6 IU/L, LH was 32.6 IU/L, prolactin was 12.9 ng/mL, and estradiol was 32 pg/mL. Her thyroid function tests were normal and her karyotype was 46 XX.

Discussion of Cases 34–36

Cases 34–36 are patients who present with primary amenorrhea, have no other associated symptoms or physical findings to suggest chromosomal abnormalities such as Turner's syndrome, and who have high gonadotropin levels. These patients have chromosomally competent gonadal failure – that is, 46 chromosomes as opposed to the 45 typical of Turner's syndrome. Abnormal formation of the gonads or abnormal migration of germ cells leads to significant early deficiency of germ cells and hence hypogonadism, usually manifested at puberty. Breast development is usually absent or minimal (as in Case 36), and infantile internal genitalia are found. As these patients have not previously been exposed to much estrogen, hot flashes do not occur. The diagnosis of primary gonadal failure is usually clearly evident from the high gonadotropin levels. Although the majority are 'female' with 46 XX karyotypes, a few are 'female' phenotypically but have XY karyotypes. In such cases (referred to as Swyer's syndrome), the internal genitalia are female (i.e. they have a uterus) because loss of testicular tissue occurred so early on that there was no production of Müllerian inhibitory substance to get rid of Müllerian structures, as occurs in a normal male with normal testes. Thus it is mandatory to obtain a karyotype in patients with chromosomally competent gonadal failure in order to rule out a Y line, as these gonads have the potential for malignant transformation and need to be removed.

Case 35 illustrates the need for early diagnosis and proper management. These patients are hypo-estrogenic throughout their lives, with all the long-term consequences of estrogen deficiency both on the cardiovascular system and on bone. Bone mineral density analysis revealed evidence of severe osteopenia and this related to estrogen deficiency over the years. According to the World Health Organization (WHO) classification, osteopenia refers to bone mass –1 to –2.5 standard deviations below peak bone mass, and osteoporosis refers to bone mass equal to or less than –2.5 SD below peak bone mass. In Case 35, it is important to ensure adequate estrogen replacement.

CHROMOSOMALLY INCOMPETENT GONADAL FAILURE (TURNER'S SYNDROME)

Case 37

A 23-year-old patient was referred for management of hormone replacement. She was complaining of vaginal dryness. Turner's syndrome was diagnosed at a very young age and gonadectomy was performed at the age of 5 years due to the presence of XY mosaicism. From the age of 8 years to 15 years, she received low-dose conjugated equine estrogen (CEE), combined with growth hormone from age 10–12 years. After the age of 15 years, she was treated with CEE, 0.625 mg daily, together with cyclic medroxyprogesterone acetate (MPA), and this was changed to low-dose oral contraceptives at the age of 19 years. She had previously been a smoker but had quit.

Examination
The patient was 4 feet 10 inches (147 cm) tall, weighed 83 lb (38 kg) and had mild cubitus valgus, pectus excavatum and a kyphotic posture. Her breasts were well developed and general and pelvic examinations did not reveal any abnormalities.

Case 38

A 27-year-old patient was seen for hormonal management. She had been diagnosed with Turner's syndrome at the age of 11 years. At the age of 22 years she had also been diagnosed with primary hypothyroidism and was given thyroid replacement therapy. She was currently on conjugated equine estrogen (CEE) 1.25 mg together with cyclic medroxyprogesterone acetate (MPA) treatment.

Examination
The patient was of short stature, and had cubitus valgus and short fourth metacarpals. Her breasts were well developed.

Laboratory Tests
Her serum TSH level was 9.1 μIU/mL (normal range 0.32–5.0 μIU/mL) and her dose of thyroxine was increased.

Case 39

An 18-year-old patient was referred for management of Turner's syndrome, which had been first diagnosed at the age of 13 years following poor growth and development. She had been given low-dose CEE (0.3 mg) and, more recently, MPA had been added in cyclic fashion, which resulted in cyclical menstrual flow. The patient had also recently been diagnosed as having aortic stenosis, and echocardiography suggested mild to moderate stenosis with mild left ventricular hypertrophy.

Examination
Her height was 4 feet 10 inches (147 cm) and her weight was 123 lb (56 kg). She had short fourth and fifth metacarpals but no other skeletal abnormalities. Her breasts were Tanner stage III. A systolic ejection murmur was audible.

Laboratory Tests
Her thyroid function tests were normal and her FSH level was 46 IU/L.

Case 40

A 37-year-old patient was referred because of primary amenorrhea. She had little breast development and had never been treated. She did not have hot flashes. Her past medical history was significant for hypertension. She had been a slow learner but showed no signs of mental retardation.

Examination
Her height was 4 feet 8 inches (142 cm) and her weight was 137 lb (62 kg). She had dry skin, a deep voice, and delayed return of ankle jerks, but no goiter. Other abnormalities included cubitus valgus, a high arched palate, shield chest, short fourth and fifth metatarsals, and slight webbing of her neck. Her breasts were Tanner stage III and pelvic examination revealed a small uterus.

Laboratory Tests
Her FSH was 45.8 IU/L, LH was 32 IU/L, prolactin was 7.4 ng/mL and estradiol was 30 pg/mL. Her TSH was 9.5 μIU/mL, and antimicrosomal antibodies were strongly positive. Her T_4 was 6.5 μg/dL, T_3 resin uptake was 27%, and her free thyroxine index was 1.8. Her karyotype was 45 XO. Bone mineral density studies showed that both her spine and her hip were at marked risk for fractures.

Discussion of Cases 37–40

Patients with Turner's syndrome may present with primary amenorrhea, although they are usually diagnosed in childhood because of poor growth and development (as in Case 39), and occasionally in early childhood with lymphedema. Rarely, they are not diagnosed until well into adult life, as in Case 40. This poses a major medical problem, as these patients are hypo-estrogenic and thus face the long-term bone and cardiovascular consequences of estrogen deficiency. In Case 40, bone mineral density (BMD) studies revealed a marked risk for osteoporosis in both spine and hip. Patients with Turner's syndrome should receive adequate amounts of estrogen, and bone status can be determined by repeat BMD studies. These patients are also at greater than average risk of developing autoimmune thyroid disease, as is illustrated by Cases 38 and 40. Although the majority of patients with Turner's syndrome are XO, some will be mosaic, usually 45 XO/46 XX, but occasionally 45 XO/46 XY. It is important to perform a karyotype in *all* patients with Turner's syndrome, since the finding of a Y line necessitates gonadectomy because these gonads are potentially premalignant. This is precisely what occurred in Case 37. Patients with Y lines do not necessarily exhibit signs of virilization, and may only be detected by karyotyping.

Coarctation of the aorta or valvular heart disease may occur in these patients (as in Case 39). Hormone replacement in these patients should include an initial period (6 months or longer) of unopposed estrogen, to allow adequate breast development, prior to the addition of progestin for endometrial protection.

The gonadal failure of these patients is manifested biochemically as high FSH, and usually also high LH, together with low estradiol levels. Lack of an X-chromosome leads to accelerated germ cell atresia. External and internal genitalia are normal, and these patients are suitable candidates for receiving donated oocytes. Their uteri are hormonally prepared, the donor oocytes are fertilized with their partners' sperm, and the resulting embryos are transferred transcervically into the uterus.

PREMATURE GONADAL FAILURE

Case 41

A 27-year-old patient attended for advice regarding amenorrhea and infertility. Her menarche occurred at age 10 years with normal menses until the age of 16 years. At this time, her periods became irregular and she was amenorrheic by her early to mid-twenties. Work-up at the age of 25 years had included a laparoscopy which showed small ovaries, and multiple courses of clomiphene had failed to induce ovulation or menses. Her past medical history was non-contributory, and there was no family history of amenorrhea.

Examination
She weighed 164 lb (75 kg) and her blood pressure was 120/84 mmHg. She was clinically euthyroid and had no goiter. Her breasts were normal and without galactorrhea, and a recent pelvic examination had been normal.

Laboratory Tests
LH was 91 IU/L, FSH was 177 IU/L, estradiol was < 20 pg/mL, prolactin was 7 ng/mL, testosterone was 48 ng/dL, DHEA-S was 122 µg/dL, thyroid function was normal and cortisol was 8 µg/dL (p.m.). Chromosomal analysis showed a 46 XX karyotype.

Case 42

A 28-year-old patient was seen who was requesting information about her fertility potential. Her menarche occurred at age 16 years. She had regular cycles and had two pregnancies at the age of 17 and 19 years, after which she took oral contraceptives until the age of 27 years. When she stopped taking the oral contraceptives, she became amenorrheic and developed hot flashes. There was no past history of radiation, chemotherapy or autoimmune disease, and no family history of premature ovarian failure.

Examination
There were no significant findings.

Laboratory Tests
FSH was 60 IU/L was estradiol and was 45 pg/mL.

Case 43

A 19-year-old patient was referred because of secondary amenorrhea. Her menarche occurred at age 14 years, and she had regular cycles until the age of 17 years. She became amenorrheic at this time and was given oral contraceptives for a short while. She remained amenorrheic while off the birth control pills. She had also experienced some hot flashes. There was no other significant personal or family history.

Examination
The patient was 6 feet 1 inch tall (185 cm) and weighed 235 lb (107 kg), and she was clinically euthyroid. Her breasts were well developed, and pelvic examination was normal.

Laboratory Tests
Her FSH was 44 IU/L, LH was 22 IU/L and estradiol was 46 pg/mL. Her TSH and prolactin levels were normal. Anti-ovarian antibodies were not detected. A karyotype was performed which showed 46 chromosomes. One X-chromosome was normal, but the second showed inversion between band q22 and q28, with some partial loss of material. No Y material was detected.

Case 44

A 38-year-old patient was seen for hormonal management. Her menarche occurred at age 15 years, and she had regular cycles. From the age of 18 to 26 years, she used oral contraceptives. She became amenorrheic at this time and was diagnosed with premature ovarian failure. There was no significant past medical or family history. She was taking conjugated equine estrogen and cyclic medroxyprogesterone acetate, and would have hot flashes if she skipped her treatment.

Examination
There were no abnormal findings.

Laboratory Tests
Thyroid function was normal. Karyotyping was suggested but was not performed.

Discussion of Cases 41–44

Case 41 presented with secondary amenorrhea and premature gonadal failure at an *early* age without obvious cause. Such cases probably represent a continuum of primary gonadal failure with primary amenorrhea, as discussed for Cases 34–36 on p. 62. In Case 41, there were some germ cells and follicles present and the patient continued to menstruate until her early twenties. It is therefore also recommended that a karyotype be performed in patients with early-onset gonadal failure and secondary amenorrhea, as there is a small possibility of picking up Y-chromosomal material. The presence of such material is indicative of the potential presence of streak testicular tissue that needs to be removed prior to malignant transformation.

Case 43 illustrates the same problem. This patient developed secondary amenorrhea at the age of 17 years, and had documented high gonadotropins levels. A karyotype was performed, and although there was no evidence of Y-chromosomal material, one of her X-chromosomes showed partial loss of material and an inversion between q22 and q28. These chromosomal abnormalities are likely to have explained her very-early-onset ovarian failure.

In Case 42, it is not possible to date the onset of the secondary amenorrhea resulting from primary gonadal failure because the patient took oral contraceptives at the age of 19 years after her second pregnancy. There was no obvious cause of gonadal failure. It is generally recommended that in the absence of an obvious cause, a karyotype should be obtained in individuals with primary gonadal failure who are under the age of 30 years. The same also applies to Case 44.

AUTOIMMUNE OVARIAN FAILURE

Case 45

A 34-year-old patient was seen because of amenorrhea. Her menarche occurred at age 11 years, followed by regular 28-day cycles. At the age of 32 years, she achieved pregnancy and was delivered by Caesarean section. Her postpartum course was complicated by a ruptured spleen and adult respiratory distress syndrome. She did not breast-feed and she remained amenorrheic postpartum. Her past medical history and family history were non-contributory. She also complained of hot flashes.

Examination
She weighed 195 lb (88.6 kg) and her blood pressure was 116/70 mmHg. She had significant vitiligo on her hands. She was clinically euthyroid and had no goiter. Breast, pelvic and general physical examinations were otherwise unremarkable.

Laboratory Tests
Thyroid function and prolactin levels were normal, estradiol was 29 pg/mL, FSH was 45.3 IU/L and cortisol was 18.8 µg/dL.

Follow-up
The patient was given hormone replacement therapy. Three years after her initial evaluation, she developed a small goiter and very positive anti-thyroglobulin antibodies (titer > 700 U/mL with normal titer up to 25 U/mL). A Cortrosyn stimulation test was performed, and her cortisol level rose from 7.3 to 28.8 µg/dL, which is a normal response.

Case 46

A 34-year-old patient was seen because of nausea, diarrhea and dizziness. She had had a diagnosis of Addison's disease from the age of 18 years and was therefore hospitalized. Investigations in hospital revealed hyperthyroidism, and the diagnosis of Graves' disease was made. After initial antithyroid medications, radioactive iodine was administered. Although her early reproductive development had been normal, she became amenorrheic by the age of 18 years and was diagnosed with premature menopause. An FSH of 62 IU/L at a subsequent date confirmed this diagnosis. She had taken conjugated equine estrogens and medroxyprogesterone acetate since the age of 18 years. A bone mineral density study at the age of 36 years revealed normal density in her hip but reduced density in her lumbar spine.

Case 47

A 32-year-old patient was referred because of irregular menses. Her menarche occurred at age 12 years, and her cycles were regular until the age of 28 years, at which time they occurred at increasing intervals, approximately every 3–5 months. There was no significant past medical history or family history. She had hot flashes at the onset of her menstrual irregularities.

Examination
She was clinically euthyroid and had no goiter. Breast, general and pelvic examination were unremarkable.

Laboratory Tests
Thyroid function tests were normal. Her prolactin level was 8.5 ng/mL, LH was 32 IU/L, FSH was 144 IU/L and estradiol was 21 pg/mL (postmenopausal range). A repeat FSH measurement was 100 IU/L. Her karyotype was 46 XX. Anti-ovarian antibodies were positive, antithyroid antibodies were negative and her serum cortisol level was 28.7 μg/dL (on oral contraceptives).

Case 48

A 41-year-old patient was seen because of secondary amenorrhea. After a normal menarche, she had established regular cycles and had undergone two pregnancies. In her late thirties she had become amenorrheic and had developed hot flashes. At the age of 38 years, her right ovary was removed because of a cyst. Her past medical history was significant for Hashimoto's thyroiditis, and she had been on thyroid hormone replacement therapy for many years.

Examination
Examination was only significant for a 40-gram smooth goiter. She was clinically euthyroid.

Laboratory Tests
As well as evidence of her menopausal state, her anti-ovarian antibodies were positive.

Discussion of Cases 45–48

Both Cases 45 and 46 had premature ovarian failure, as determined by failure of ovarian function prior to the age of 40 years. In Case 46, this occurred in the patient's late teens and she became amenorrheic in the setting of diagnoses of Addison's disease and Graves' disease. Both of these conditions have autoimmune etiologies. In Graves' disease, the production of thyroid-stimulating antibodies leads to stimulation of thyroid function and hence hyperthyroidism. In Addison's disease, the antibodies are directed against enzymes involved in steroidogenesis, and glucocorticoid and mineralocorticoid deficiency follow the destruction of adrenal tissue. Ovarian failure with lymphocytic infiltration of the ovaries and destruction of ovarian tissue can also occur as part of the same polyglandular autoimmune process, again with antibodies directed against enzymes in the steroidogenic cascade. Other autoimmune diseases, such as hypoparathyroidism, systemic lupus and rheumatoid arthritis, may also be seen in these patients and their families. It is important to replace estrogen deficiency adequately in these young patients, who may otherwise suffer significant bone loss. This is particularly important in the face of glucocorticoid replacement, hyperthyroidism or replacement therapy for hypothyroidism, as excess glucocorticoids or thyroxine may also contribute to bone loss.

In Case 45, the cause of premature ovarian failure was not initially apparent, and anti-ovarian antibodies were not determined (and may indeed be absent after the initial process). However, the vitiligo found in this patient was suggestive of an autoimmune process. Patients with possible autoimmune disease or those with premature ovarian failure of undetermined cause should periodically be tested for the possibility of hypothyroidism (measurement of thyroid function with T_4, T_3 resin uptake and TSH, and antithyroid antibodies which can be directed against either thyroglobulin or the thyroid peroxidase enzyme – previously known as anti-microsomal antibodies). They should also be tested for the possibility of Addison's disease. For this purpose, a screening Cortrosyn test is utilized. Cortrosyn contains the active portion of the ACTH molecule; 250 µg are given intravenously and serum cortisol levels are measured at baseline and after 30 and 60 minutes. A rise in serum cortisol exceeding 7 µg/dL (e.g. from 6 to 15 µg/dL) or a peak cortisol value equal to or exceeding 18 µg/dL is consistent with normal adrenal function.

Cases 47 and 48 also had premature ovarian failure. In both of these patients anti-ovarian antibodies were demonstrated, which are highly suggestive of autoimmune destruction of ovarian tissue. Case 48 already exhibited another autoimmune disease, namely Hashimoto's thyroiditis.

CHEMOTHERAPY/IRRADIATION-INDUCED OVARIAN FAILURE

Case 49

A 37-year-old patient attended to discuss her fertility potential. Her reproductive history was as follows. Her menarche occurred at age 11 years, and she had regular menses and a pregnancy at the age of 25 years. This was followed by normal menses. At the age of 35 years, colorectal cancer was diagnosed and she was given chemotherapy with 5 fluorouracil and also received approximately 5000 cGy of pelvic irradiation. She became amenorrheic and was treated with estrogen and subsequently with estradiol pellets, together with a progestin. The only additional history was that of hypothyroidism, for which she was receiving treatment.

Examination
The patient was clinically euthyroid and had no goiter. General examination was unremarkable. Pelvic examination revealed a small uterus and no adnexal enlargement.

Case 50

A 24-year-old patient attended to discuss her future fertility potential. Hodgkin's lymphoma had been diagnosed at the age of 11 years, and she received six courses of mechlorethamine hydrochloride, vincristine, prednisone and procarbazine (MOPP), together with irradiation of her neck and chest. She had oophoropexy in anticipation of abdominal irradiation, but was never irradiated below the diaphragm. After these treatments, by the age of 14 years, she had developed breasts, and menses were induced by oral contraceptives which she took until the age of 17 years. After discontinuing these pills, her menses were irregular but, despite this, she achieved pregnancy. She had a miscarriage and resumed more regular cycles until the time of her visit at the age of 24 years.

Examination
The patient was clinically euthyroid and had no goiter. General and pelvic examinations did not reveal any abnormalities.

Laboratory Tests
Early-cycle LH was 1.2 IU/L, FSH was 4.9 IU/L and mid-luteal progesterone was 14 ng/mL.

Case 51

A 30-year-old patient attended to discuss her reproductive situation. She developed life-threatening vasculitis at the age of 23 years, and was treated with large doses of glucocorticoids for several years. This treatment was more recently switched to cyclophosphamide and at the time of her visit her cumulative dose of cyclophosphamide was 15 g. Her menarche occurred at age 10 years, followed by regular cycles. Over the course of treatment with cyclophosphamide, she missed a few menstrual cycles and her flow diminished. She had no hot flashes or other symptoms at the time of her visit.

Examination
Examination was normal and the patient did not attend for laboratory tests.

Case 52

A 21-year-old patient was referred because of secondary amenorrhea and increased body and facial hair. Her menarche occurred at age 12 years, and she had continued to have regular menstrual cycles until the age of 16 years. At this time, Ewing's sarcoma was diagnosed and she was given chemotherapy – she received adriamycin, etoposide, taxol and ifosfamide (a synthetic analogue of cyclophosphamide). She became oligomenorrheic/amenorrheic after her first course of chemotherapy.

Examination
The patient had complete scalp hair loss and some excess body hair. Pelvic examination was normal.

Laboratory Tests
FSH was 128 IU/L, LH was 40.7 IU/L, estradiol was 60 pg/mL, prolactin was 13.3 ng/mL, testosterone was 93 ng/mL and DHEA-S was 249 μg/dL. Thyroid function tests were normal.

Discussion of Cases 49–52

Both radiation and chemotherapy have profound effects on gonadal function by destroying germ cells. A woman is only endowed with a finite number of germ cells, and she has no mechanism for renewal. Germ cells are lost by the process of atresia during the reproductive years and, when they become exhausted in the late forties or early fifties, menopause is said to occur with its attendant symptoms of hot flashes, night sweats, etc., indicative of estrogen deficiency. Amenorrhea or oligomenorrhea in the context of chemotherapy and abdominal/pelvic radiation as in Case 49 is thus almost always related to a process of premature ovarian failure. Serum gonadotropins, especially FSH, will be elevated and serum estradiol levels will be low. As germ cells are continually lost during the reproductive years, it follows that premature ovarian failure is more likely to occur in older women than in younger individuals. For example, the cumulative dose of cyclophosphamide that usually results in amenorrhea in a 20-year-old is approximately 20 g, in a 30-year-old it is 10 g and in a 40-year-old it is 5 g. In case 51, where the patient was 30 years old, a cumulative dose of 15 g had caused menstrual irregularities. Of the various chemotherapeutic agents employed, alkylating agents are the most likely to cause germ cell loss. It appears that the prepubertal gonad is somewhat protected against the damaging effects of chemotherapy and irradiation. For example, despite six courses of mechlorethamine hydrochloride, vincristine, prednisone and procarbazine (MOPP) Case 50, who received treatment at the age of 11 years, established spontaneous menses and had normal gonadotropin levels and was ovulating when she was seen at the age of 24 years. Oophoropexy is sometimes performed in young women who are about to receive pelvic irradiation. In this procedure, the ovaries are displaced so that they lie further away from the field of radiation.

Case 52 concerns a young woman who developed premature ovarian failure at the age of 16–17 years, following chemotherapy, and who had documented elevated gonadotropin levels. Loss of scalp hair was related to this therapy, but increased body and facial hair was related to excess androgen. Her testosterone levels were elevated and this increase was probably predominantly of ovarian origin. Although germ cells may be destroyed by the chemotherapy, the ovarian stroma remains active and can continue to produce androgens.

PREMENSTRUAL SYNDROME

Case 53

A 42-year-old patient was referred because of mood changes, irritability, fluid retention and headaches. These symptoms occurred predominantly premenstrually, and were increasing in severity with time. Her menarche occurred at age 13 years, and although her cycles were not very regular, she had achieved pregnancy three times. During the previous few years, her cycles had actually been more regular. She had tried oral contraceptives for a short while, but these gave her headaches and caused further fluid retention, so she stopped taking them.

Examination
She was clinically euthyroid and mildly hirsute, but otherwise the examination was negative.

Laboratory Tests
Her thyroid function tests were normal. Her FSH (early cycle) was 4.7 IU/L, prolactin was 6.3 ng/mL, testosterone was 21 ng/dL and DHEA-S was 131 µg/dL.

Discussion of Case 53

Premenstrual syndrome is the cyclic appearance of symptoms occurring prior to menses and interfering with the patient's lifestyle or work. The symptoms of this patient were among the commonest; others include depression, breast tenderness, food cravings and anxiety. Theories of etiology include low progesterone levels, falling estrogen concentrations, increased renin or angiotensin activity, endogenous opioid withdrawal and response to prostaglandins. However, no significant discernible differences have been consistently demonstrated between individuals with and without symptoms. Recent evidence suggests that there may be aberrant brain sensitivity to normal hormonal profiles in patients with this syndrome.

Treatment has been largely empiric, and includes the use of diuretics such as spironolactone, oral contraceptives, vitamin B_6, progesterone supplementation and prostaglandin-synthesis inhibitors, which may help to relieve dysmenorrhea and headaches. The use of antidepressants such as fluoxetine and sertraline and anxiolytics such as alprazolam has also been successful in some patients. Medical (using gonadotropin-releasing hormone agonists with add-back estrogen-progestin) and surgical oophorectomy has also been successful, but should only be used as a last resort.

Preview of Cases 54–72

The following 19 cases concern patients with polycystic ovary syndrome and androgen excess disorders. Hyperandrogenism is the commonest endocrinopathy of women of reproductive age, affecting approximately 6% of them. It is also a multi-faceted disorder. To cover this important topic, a brief overview will be given, followed by the actual cases, which are grouped together in smaller sections, each followed by a discussion.

In 1935, Stein and Leventhal described the association between amenorrhea or irregular menses, hirsutism, and enlarged cystic ovaries. Despite over 50 years of progress, this remains one of the most controversial and enigmatic areas of repro-ductive endocrinology. The terms hyperandrogenism, chronic anovulation and polycystic ovary syndrome have been used interchangeably to refer to the constel-lation of symptoms and signs that are characteristic of this condition. The symptoms are those of (1) hyperandrogenism (namely hirsutism, acne, oily skin and hair, and male-pattern baldness), (2) ovulatory disturbances (namely irregular menses, amenorrhea and dysfunctional uterine bleeding) and (3) obesity (in particular, central or abdominal obesity is often (but not always) associated with this condition. The clinical, biochemical and pathologic features are outlined in Box 3.1. Plate 3.1 shows a polycystic ovary with thickened capsule, multiple subcapsular cysts and stromal hyperplasia. Pathophysiologically, this condition may arise through disturbances of diverse mechanisms, and thus the term polycystic ovary syndrome (PCOS) is an appropriate one and will be used throughout the remainder of this discussion.

Androgens are produced both by the ovaries and by the adrenal glands. Testosterone, which is the potent androgenic product of these two glands, is also derived from the peripheral conversion of androstenedione (another androgen that is produced by both glands). However it is derived, testosterone is converted at its site of action (e.g. the skin) to a more potent androgen dihydrotestosterone via a local enzyme 5α-reductase. In the adrenal gland (and to a much lesser extent in the ovary), dehydroepiandrosterone (DHEA), a weak androgen, is also produced. This compound may undergo sulfation to DHEA-S, and this occurs virtually exclusively in the adrenal glands. For practical purposes, therefore, serum DHEA-S reflects adrenal androgen production, whereas total serum testosterone (which is to a large extent bound to sex-hormone-binding globulin) reflects ovarian or adrenal androgen production. The clinical symptoms of hirsutism, acne (sebum production is androgen related) and alopecia reflect increased production, increased local 5α-reductase activity and local sensitivity. The presence or absence of hirsutism may also relate to the number and distribution of hair follicles. For example, East Asian females seldom manifest hirsutism because of the lower numbers of hair follicles per unit area of skin.

A state of hyperandrogenism (HA) is central to the pathophysiology of PCOS. The HA explains the clinical symptoms of hirsutism, acne and alopecia. The excess

---

Box 3.1 The clinical, biochemical and pathologic features of PCOS

Clinical features
1 Menstrual irregularities, usually dating from the menarche
2 Hyperandrogenism – hirsutism, acne, alopecia, oily skin and hair
3 Obesity – usually android (abdominal)

Biochemical features
1 High androgens – testosterone and/or androstenedione and/or DHEA-S
2 High LH:FSH ratio
3 Low sex-hormone-binding globulin (mediated by high androgens and insulin-resistant state)
4 High estrogen state, as evidenced by withdrawal bleeding following medroxyprogesterone acetate
5 Insulin resistance, manifested as acanthosis nigricans and/or elevated fasting or postprandial serum insulin levels in the presence of normal or elevated glucose levels
6 High prolactin – in about 20% of cases; it may be episodic

Pathologic features
1 Thickened ovarian capsule (androgen mediated)
2 Multiple subcortical cysts giving rosary-like appearance (seen on ultrasound examination)
3 Stromal hyperplasia

---

androgens are peripherally (predominantly in adipose tissue) converted to estrogens (predominantly to estrone) via peripheral aromatase. The excess estrogens interfere with normal ovarian/gonadotropin feedback, leading to inadequate FSH activity and hence stagnated folliculogenesis (no mature Graafian follicle, but numerous immature follicles or cysts – hence the term 'polycystic'). As a dominant follicle is not produced, there is no luteal phase, and therefore a state of chronic anovulation prevails. The endometrial lining of the uterus thus responds to unopposed estrogens. The result of this chronic estrogen exposure may be amenorrhea or oligomenorrhea, with the occasional estrogen breakthrough bleeding. There may also be dysfunctional uterine bleeding which may consist of constant spotting or uncontrolled flow, (heavy or prolonged), due to erratic breakdown of an unstable endometrium. Occasionally the patient ovulates, usually with a prolonged follicular phase and a short, inadequate luteal phase.

The origin of the obesity that frequently accompanies PCOS is poorly understood. What is clear, however, is that obesity exacerbates the pathologic derangements of this syndrome. For example, excess adipose tissue allows for increased peripheral aromatization of androgens to estrogens. It has been clearly demonstrated that weight loss may improve or lessen the manifestations of PCOS, (e.g. resulting in less ovulatory disturbances). Obesity is also related to the insulin resistance characteristic of this syndrome (see discussion below).

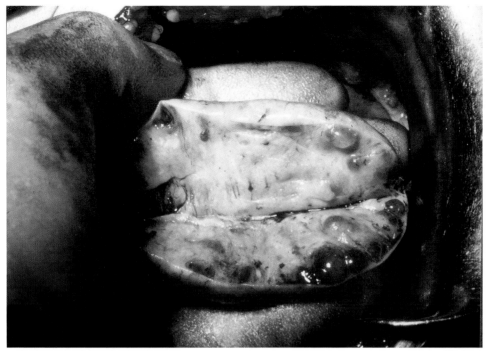

PLATE 3.1 Polycystic ovary syndrome: Cut surface of ovary.

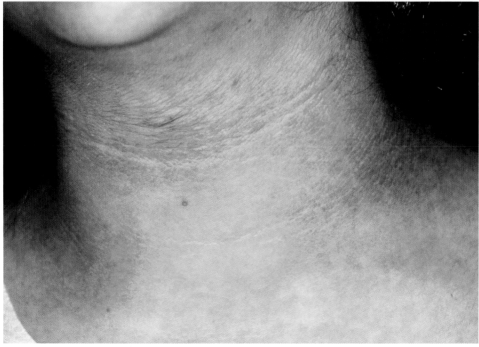

PLATE 3.2 Young girl with acanthosis nigricans and hirsutism.

The question of the origin of the androgens (ovary vs. adrenal) has also been the subject of much debate. In reality, the excess androgens may arise from one or both glands (see Box 3.2). The question of why *adrenal* hyperandrogenism should lead to polycystic *ovaries* has also been raised. Again, in reality, it may do so. For example, patients with Cushing's syndrome may have PCOS, as may patients with late-onset congenital adrenal hyperplasia (21-hydroxylase deficiency, which is an adrenal enzyme deficiency) or androgen-producing adrenal tumors. Even when adrenal androgens are clearly elevated, as in Cushing's syndrome, the ovary may also be a secondary source of excess androgens. This may occur at least in part because the hormonal disturbances often lead to elevated LH concentrations (in contrast to the decreased FSH activity; see further discussion below). LH drives the ovarian theca and stroma to produce androgens, and hence a vicious cycle is set up. Finally, with regard to adrenal HA, most patients with evidence of excess adrenal HA do not have Cushing's syndrome, late-onset congenital adrenal hyperplasia or adrenal tumors. During and after adrenarche, the adrenal glands respond to pituitary ACTH to produce androgens, and the capacity to respond, both in terms of the biochemical response to graduated doses of ACTH and in terms of the *amount of adrenal tissue* that is capable of responding, may vary between individuals. Thus some young women may produce excessive amounts of adrenal androgens.

Box 3.2 Sources of serum androgens in women

1 *Testosterone*:
   25% ovarian, 25% adrenal source
   50% from peripheral conversion of androstenedione

2 *Androstenedione*:
   50% ovarian, 50% adrenal source

3 *Dehydroepiandrosterone (DHEA)*:
   90% adrenal, 10% ovarian source

4 *Dehydroepiandrosterone sulfate (DHEA-S)*:
   100% adrenal source

It is also clear that in many cases – and probably the majority – the ovary is the predominant or exclusive source of androgen excess. In the context of ovarian hyperandrogenism, it is now apparent (and currently the major focus of PCOS research) that states of insulin resistance are integrally linked to ovarian hyperandrogenism. Insulin resistance may result not only from rare syndromes affecting insulin binding (type A) and anti-insulin receptor antibodies (type B), but also from much more common and probably genetically related defects of insulin action, usually at post-receptor level (type C). Obesity, a common accompaniment, is well known to exacerbate insulin resistance further. Insulin resistance, in the presence of a viable functional pancreas, leads to a state of hyperinsulinemia, which can result in acanthosis nigricans, namely raised vellus areas of pigmentation normally seen in the back of the neck and axillae. Excess insulin in the presence of gonadotropins such as LH can also stimulate the ovarian stroma and theca to produce androgens, acting via its own receptors or via insulin-like growth factor I receptors in the ovary. The resulting hyperandrogenism will respond to either gonadotropin suppression (as with the use of oral contraceptives or analogues of gonadotropin-releasing hormone) or agents that lower insulin levels by improving insulin action (e.g. metformin and thiazolidinediones). There is also evidence that androgens themselves may impair insulin action and may thus set up a vicious cycle.

Obesity is present in over 50% of PCOS patients. As indicated above, it exacerbates the clinical manifestations of PCOS. It is also now apparent that all forms of obesity are not equal in their metabolic effects. Android obesity with a high waist-to-hip ratio (as opposed to gluteofemoral or gynoid obesity, with a lower ratio) is excess fat in the abdominal location, and is associated with higher degrees of insulin resistance. Obese PCOS patients are commonly android, which may in part explain their greater degree of insulin resistance compared to obese controls. Although there may be a genetic predisposition to androidness, there is also evidence that androgens may mediate deposition of fat in abdominal locations, further exacerbating insulin resistance.

One of the most important laboratory hallmarks of PCOS is an elevated LH with a high LH:FSH ratio (a ratio of 3 is virtually pathognomomic). The cause of this disparity in gonadotropins is the subject of much controversy. It may be mediated in part by estrogens and possibly by non-steroidal hormones such as inhibin (or similar substances). It has also recently been shown that high LH levels may result from hyperinsulinemia. Although the available evidence suggests that the 'inappropriate' gonadotropin secretion of PCOS is a result of the hormonal disturbances, there is also a school of thought which suggests that the primary abnormality of PCOS may be central – that is, originating in the brain and altering the pituitary response to GNRH in favor of LH. Studies of chronobiology in relation to LH have suggested this hypothesis. Although it is possible that in some patients the etiology of PCOS may be centrally mediated, this is clearly not so in all cases. These two possibilities are depicted in Figure 3.1.

PCOS is managed according to the predominant symptom and pathophysiology. Table 3.1 outlines the management strategies used in patients with PCOS and their mechanisms of action. Oral contraceptives are often used to reduce hyperandrogenism, protect the endometrium from hyperplasia and cancer and alleviate dysfunctional bleeding. Spironolactone may be used in conjunction with oral contraceptives, acting as an androgen blocker at target tissues. Glucocorticoids reduce adrenal hyperandrogenism and have been shown to improve acne and ovulatory efficiency when used in such cases. Metformin, acting predominantly on the liver, improves insulin action, reduces circulating insulin concentrations and thereby reduces ovarian androgen synthesis. The improvement in hormonal status also improves ovulatory efficiency. Thiazolidinediones also have an overall action

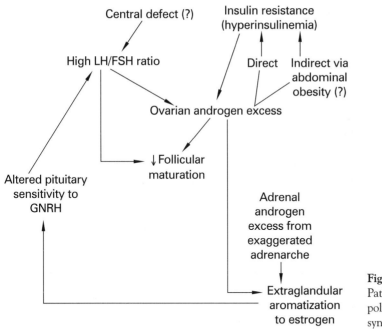

Central defect (?)

Insulin resistance
(hyperinsulinemia)

High LH/FSH ratio

Direct   Indirect via
abdominal
obesity (?)

Ovarian androgen excess

Altered pituitary
sensitivity to
GNRH

↓ Follicular
maturation

Adrenal
androgen
excess from
exaggerated
adrenarche

Extraglandular
aromatization
to estrogen

Figure 3.1
Pathophysiology of
polycystic ovary
syndrome.

similar to that of metformin, although their site of action in improving insulin sensitivity is predominantly on muscle. Concerns about liver toxicity dictate extreme caution, and these drugs are not currently approved for this purpose. Clomiphene citrate, acting as an anti-estrogen at the hypothalamic level, increases GNRH and therefore LH and FSH availability and thus promotes ovulation in many individuals with PCOS. Doses of up to 200 mg daily (given for 5 days in the early cycle) may be required, and a significant percentage of PCOS patients are resistant to even these high doses. In such patients, the addition of metformin or thiazolidinediones has often resulted in ovulation, even when using much lower doses of clomiphene citrate. Pure FSH, injected subcutaneously or intramuscularly, is approved for ovulation induction in clomiphene-resistant PCOS subjects. Since these individuals have a significant risk for both multiple gestation and severe hyperstimulation syndrome, they must be carefully monitored using serial ultrasound and estradiol determinations during each course of treatment. Only physicians familiar with such monitoring should supervise this treatment.

Table 3.1 Mechanism of action of treatments for PCOS

Treatment	Mechanism of action
Oral contraceptives	Reduce LH and its stimulation of ovarian thecal/stromal androgen synthesis Increase sex-hormone-binding globulin (SHBG), reduce free androgens Protect against endometrial hyperplasia Reduce dysfunction bleeding and abnormal flow
Spironolactone[a]	Anti-androgenic action at target tissue (skin) due to competitive binding to androgen receptors Also weak inhibitor of testosterone biosynthesis
Glucocorticoids	Reduce ACTH and therefore adrenal androgen synthesis
Metformin[b]	Insulin sensitizer leading to reduced insulin concentrations and therefore less ovarian androgen production Increases SHBG, lowering free androgens
Thiazolidinediones[b]	Insulin sensitizer leading to reduced insulin concentrations and therefore less ovarian androgen production Increase SHBG, lowering free androgens
Clomiphene citrate	Activates the hypothalamic–pituitary axis, increasing availability of gonadotropins, LH and FSH. Increased available FSH then drives ovarian folliculogenesis
Pure FSH	Injectable FSH is available for clomiphene-resistant patients. Risks of multiple gestation and severe hyperstimulation syndrome are significant, and appropriate monitoring with estradiol and ultrasound evaluations is mandatory

[a]Other anti-androgens, such as cyproterone acetate, are available in Europe. Flutamide is used infrequently because of concerns about liver toxicity.
[b]Both metformin and thiazolidinediones have been shown to improve ovulatory efficiency, too, but concerns about their use in pregnancy dictate careful monitoring.

POLYCYSTIC OVARY SYNDROME

Case 54

A 19-year-old patient was seen because of amenorrhea, weight gain and hirsutism. Her menarche occurred at age 17 years, and her menses had been irregular. She took oral contraceptives for a few months and resumed her irregular menses on discontinuing them. Her last period had been 5 months previously.

Examination
Her weight was 151 lb (68.6 kg) and she was mildly hirsute over her upper lip, chin and abdomen. She was not cushingoid, and a general physical examination and pelvic examinations were unremarkable. She was clinically euthyroid.

Laboratory Tests
Thyroid function tests were normal. Her LH was 13.3 IU/L, FSH was 5.2 IU/L, prolactin was 10.9 ng/mL, testosterone was 66 ng/dL and DHEA-S was 80.3 µg/dL. Her urinary free cortisol level was 28.8 µg/24 hours (normal range < 100 µg/24 hours).

Case 55

A 25-year-old patient was referred because of oligomenorrhea/amenorrhea. Her menarche occurred at age 10 years, and she had essentially regular cycles but would skip the occasional one. After the age of 15 years she became more irregular, with occasional amenorrhea of approximately 6 months' duration. Since the age of 17 years she had noticed increased body hair growth and she had gained approximately 100 lb (45 kg) in weight. Her family history was significant for diabetes (mother and grandmother) and also for hirsutism (sister).

Examination
She was overweight at 238 lb (108 kg) and had obvious acanthosis nigricans over her neck and axillae (Plate 3.2), and she was clinically euthyroid. She was severely hirsute over her face, abdomen and perineal region. She had no galactorrhea. Pelvic examination revealed a prominent clitoris.

Laboratory Tests
Her testosterone level was 193 ng/dL, her DHEA-S was 70 μg/dL and her prolactin level was 12 ng/mL. Her thyroid function tests were normal.

Case 56

A 21-year-old patient was referred because of secondary amenorrhea. Her menarche occurred at age 15 years, she was never regular and by the age of 18 years she was amenorrheic. Her other major problem was extreme obesity. She weighed 250 lb (113.6 kg) at the age of 15 years and had continued to gain weight since that time. There was a history of previous acne. She also gave a family history of obesity and non-insulin-dependent diabetes mellitus.

Examination
Her weight was 341 lb (155 kg) and her blood pressure was 120/90 mmHg. She was euthyroid and had no goiter. There was no galactorrhea but mild perineal hirsutism. She also had acanthosis nigricans over her neck. Pelvic examination was unremarkable.

Laboratory Tests
Thyroid function tests were normal. Her fasting insulin level was 37.7 μU/mL (normal range < 20 μU/mL) with a normal glycosylated hemoglobin level of 5.1%. Her testosterone level was 46 ng/dL, DHEA-S was 240 μg/dL and prolactin was 16.4 ng/mL.

Case 57

A 19-year-old patient was referred because of a history of primary amenorrhea. Breast, pubic and axillary hair development had occurred normally by the age of 13 years. At the age of 16 years, she had been given an injection of progesterone in oil, this being followed by a period. Oral contraceptives were given for a short time, but she remained amenorrheic when not taking them.

Examination
She was slightly overweight at 143 lb (65 kg), and was moderately to severely hirsute. Her clitoris was prominent and there was acanthosis in the perineal region.

Laboratory Tests
Her thyroid function was normal, LH was 4.5 IU/L, FSH was 5 IU/L, prolactin was 9 ng/mL, testosterone was 170 ng/dL (a repeat test was 93 ng/dL) and DHEA-S was 178 μg/dL. An insulin level measured 7 hours post-prandially was 71 μU/mL (normal range 0–20 μU/mL), together with a glucose level of 77 mg/dL

Follow-up
A course of birth control pills containing 50 μg ethinyl estradiol was administered, which lowered the testosterone level to < 20 ng/dL.

Case 58

A 31-year-old patient attended because of primary infertility and secondary amenorrhea. Menarche occurred at the age of 11 years, followed initially by regular cycles. By the age of 14 years they were irregular, and she became amenorrheic by the age of 17 years. She was occasionally given medroxyprogesterone acetate and would always have withdrawal menses. Clomiphene citrate treatment had failed to induce ovulation. She was seen at the age of 30 years for spotting and bleeding following intercourse. Dilatation and curettage was performed which revealed a well-differentiated adenocarcinoma of the endometrium. Laparoscopy at this time revealed polycystic ovaries.

Laboratory Tests
Her testosterone level was 113 ng/dL, DHEA-S was 370 μg/dL and prolactin was 3 ng/mL.

Discussion of Cases 54–58

Case 54 had a history of irregular menses dating from the menarche. She also complained of weight gain and was hirsute. Her high LH:FSH ratio and mildly elevated testosterone level (and the exclusion of other causes of amenorrhea such as major prolactin disturbances and Cushing's syndrone) were typical of PCOS. Cases 55 and 56 are obvious examples of ovarian hyperandrogenism associated with insulin resistance, as evidenced by the acanthosis nigricans. Case 55 had a very high testosterone level and exhibited clitoromegaly. The family history of diabetes supported the genetic propensity towards insulin resistance, certainly aggravated by the 100 lb (45 kg) weight gain. Case 56 demonstrated significant fasting hyperinsulinemia but much milder androgen excess.

Case 57 had a less common presentation of this common problem, namely primary amenorrhea. She was clearly hyperandrogenic and hyperinsulinemic. Her menstrual response to progesterone indicated adequate estrogen exposure of the endometrium. Her very high testosterone level of 170 ng/dL was also a cause for concern. Its reduction following gonadotropin suppression with the birth control pill was reassuring and rendered the possibility of tumor-mediated hyperandrogenism much less likely. Case 58 also manifested another uncommon event in this common disease, namely adenocarcinoma of the endometrium, a potential long-term result of unopposed estrogen stimulation.

Case 59

Two identical twins aged 13 years were seen because of menstrual irregularities. They were originally referred to a dermatologist because of acne and skin pigmentation, which was determined to be acanthosis nigricans. Their menarche had occurred at age 11 years, and their menses were irregular and with prolonged flow. There was a family history of diabetes mellitus (a grandmother and an aunt).

Examination

Both twins had extensive acanthosis nigricans affecting their neck, back and axillae. Both also had acne and were mildly hirsute. They were obese, weighing 191 lb (87 kg) and 224 lb (102 kg), respectively. Their waist-to-hip ratios were 0.84 and 0.87, respectively, and they had no clitoromegaly.

Table 3.2 Endocrine profiles of identical twins with acanthosis nigricans

Laboratory Test	Twin A	Twin B
Glucose (6-hour fasting)	80 mg/dL	76 mg/dL
Insulin (6-hour fasting)	93 μU/dL	84 μU/dL (normal range < 20 μU/dL)
Glycohemoglobin	5.7%	5.5 % (normal range < 6.7%)
DHEA-S	317 μg/dL	355 μg/dL
FSH	2.7 IU/L	2.6 IU/L
LH	8.1 IU/L	5.7 IU/L
Prolactin	10.9 ng/mL	8.1 ng/mL
Testosterone	51 ng/dL	54 ng/dL
Thyroid function tests	Normal	Normal

Case 60

A 12-year-old patient with severe acanthosis nigricans was referred for reproductive evaluation. Her childhood development had been normal. Adrenarche occurred at age 9.5 years and breast development at age 10.5 years. Her menarche occurred at age 11 years, and for 2 months she experienced continuous bleeding. This was followed by irregular menses, but in the few months prior to her visit they had become more regular. She had had acne since the age of 10 years. Her acanthosis had been developing for 2 years and was increasing.

Examination
Her weight was 179 lb (81 kg), her blood pressure was 120/80 mmHg, and she had very severe acanthosis affecting her neck, axillae, abdominal area and perineum. She was euthyroid and had no goiter. Her breasts were Tanner stage IV. She had moderate acne and also hirsutism affecting her thighs and perineum. There was some degree of clitoromegaly.

Laboratory Tests
Glucose was 94 mg/dL (fasting), insulin was 140.8 μU/mL (normal range 5–20 μU/mL) (see Table 3.3), glycohemoglobin was 6.7% (normal range 4–8%), LH was 8.2 IU/L, FSH was 3.1 IU/L, testosterone was 87 ng/dL, DHEA-S was 88 μg/dL, the sedimentation rate was 21 mm/hour, triglyceride was 190 mg/dL, cholesterol was 132 mg/dL and HDL was 25 mg/dL. Her progesterone level was 0.4 ng/mL 8 days prior to menses. An oral glucose tolerance test was performed.

Table 3.3 Oral glucose tolerance test

	Glucose (mg/dL)	Insulin (μU/mL)
Fasting	85	47.6
1 hour	121	>240
2 hour	110	>240
3 hour	74	125.4

Case 61

A 17-year-old African-American patient was referred because of amenorrhea and hirsutism. Her menarche occurred at age 12 years, and her menses were irregular. She took oral contraceptives from time to time, and achieved pregnancy at the age of 13 years following non-compliance. Her menses continued irregularly post-partum until the age of 16 years, when she received an injection of Depo-Provera. She remained amenorrheic when she was seen 8 months later. During the year preceding her visit, she had noted increasing hirsutism and skin pigmentation. In addition, there was an 80-lb (36-kg) weight gain.

Examination
Her weight was 217½ lb (99 kg) and her height was 5 feet 6 inches (165 cm). She was euthyroid. There was generalized acanthosis nigricans involving her neck, back, axillae and other areas, and she had moderate facial hirsutism. Pelvic examination revealed clitoromegaly.

Laboratory Tests
Her thyroid function tests were normal, her prolactin level was 8.7 ng/mL, LH was 6 IU/L and FSH was 3.1 IU/L. Her testosterone level was 336 ng/dL and her DHEA-S level was 47.3 µg/dL. Ultrasound examination of her pelvis revealed a normal uterus with normal-sized ovaries. No adnexal masses were seen.

Case 62

A 26-year-old patient was referred because of amenorrhea and infertility. Her menarche occurred at age 13 years. She was always irregular and would skip up to a few months at a time. At age 15 years, she received oral contraceptives and continued on these until 6 months prior to her visit. She had had no menses since, and a pregnancy test was negative. There was no history of acne, hirsutism, galactorrhea or hot flashes. However, she had gained 30 lb (13.6 kg) since the age of 18 years. Her mother also had irregular menses and both grandmothers had diabetes mellitus. She had had no infertility work-up.

Examination
She weighed 221 lb (100 kg) and had marked acanthosis nigricans over her neck and axillae. She was not clinically hirsute and was euthyroid. Pelvic examination did not reveal any abnormalities.

Laboratory Tests
Thyroid function was normal. Testosterone was 40.4 ng/dL, DHEA-S was 90.7 µg/dL and prolactin was 8.1 ng/mL.

Further Course
Semen analysis and postcoital tests were normal. She failed to ovulate on up to 200 mg of clomiphene citrate. Ovulation was induced once with pure FSH and human chorionic gonadotropin. She failed to achieve pregnancy and a laparoscopy was performed which revealed normal pelvic findings and patent tubes. She achieved pregnancy on the second cycle of ovulation induction using pure FSH, and delivered triplets by Caesarean section.

Discussion of Cases 59–62

Case 59 concerns a set of identical twins, both of whom presumably shared genes for insulin resistance. They had acne, extensive acanthosis nigricans, high waist-to-hip ratios and a family history of diabetes. Case 60 illustrates extreme insulin resistance to oral glucose challenge, and may represent a type A defect. She also manifested mild hypertriglyceridemia and a low HDL cholesterol level (see discussion below). Case 61 also demonstrates extreme hyperandrogenism suggestive of an ovarian tumor. Her ultrasound was normal, rendering the possibility of an ovarian tumor unlikely.

Case 62 manifested the anovulation of PCOS, and the weight gain but not the signs and symptoms of hyperandrogenism *per se*. Clomiphene stimulation failed, a not infrequent occurrence in this patient population, and she required gonadotropin stimulation. It is difficult to induce unifollicular ovulation in these patients, and they are at substantial risk of multiple gestation or severe hyperstimulation syndrome during which the ovaries enlarge, become cystic and there is general hyperemia with ascites, loss of intravascular volume and potential thromboembolic complications. This patient eventually had triplets, although she did not become pregnant on the first attempt at inducing ovulation.

Case 63

A 17-year-old patient was referred because of irregular menses. Her menarche occurred at age 15 years, and she had only had sporadic menses over the ensuing 2 years. There was no history of hirsutism or galactorrhea, but she was taking tetracyclines for treatment of acne. In addition, she gave a history of excessive exercise since age 13, although the level of activity had varied over time. There was no history of weight loss or eating disorder.

Examination
She was clinically euthyroid and had no goiter. She had mild acne but no hirsutism. There was no galactorrhea, and pelvic examination was normal.

Laboratory Tests
Her LH was 8.1 IU/L, FSH was 5 IU/L, prolactin was 11.4 ng/mL, TSH was 1.6 µIU/mL, testosterone was 41.9 ng/dL, and DHEA-S was 200.5 µg/dL.

Case 64

A 22-year-old patient was referred because of irregular menses/amenorrhea. Her menarche occurred at age 13 years, and her menses were irregular, occurring every 2–7 weeks. This continued until the age of 17 years, when she started to take oral contraceptives. Over the next 5 years she took oral contraceptives from time to time, her menses always being irregular when she was not taking them. When she attended, she had been amenorrheic for 5 months. Her past history was significant for intensive exercise from age 13 to 17 years, involving several hours of high-intensity activity per day. Since the age of 17 years she had been much less active, although occasionally she would resume running several miles per day. In addition, she had been bulimic for 10 years and her weight fluctuated fairly widely. She had also had acne since being a teenager.

Examination
She weighed 165 lb (75 kg) and her height was 5 feet 10 inches (178 cm). She was clinically euthyroid and had no goiter. She had acne but no hirsutism, and there was no galactorrhea. Pelvic examination was normal.

Laboratory Tests
Her thyroid function tests, including TSH, were normal. Her LH was 10.7 IU/L, FSH was 4.7 IU/L, prolactin was 6.3 ng/mL, testosterone was 55 ng/dL, DHEA-S was 127 μg/dL, and estradiol was 42 pg/mL.

Discussion of Cases 63 and 64

Cases 63 and 64 represent diagnostic challenges. Both patients presented with a history of menstrual disturbances since menarche, but also had a history of acne. Both also gave a history of excessive exercise, but this history was sporadic and not persistent. Case 64 even had an eating disorder (bulimia), although she had never been very thin. The possibility of a functional hypothalamic disorder (as seen with exercise and weight loss) was certainly entertained. However, neither patient resumed normal menses during times of limited exercise. Both had mild acne and no hirsutism. Laboratory tests did not support a hypothalamic disorder in either case. Case 64 had a high LH:FSH ratio (> 2) and a high testosterone level. Case 63 had borderline elevated testosterone, and although her LH level was high normal, the LH:FSH ratio was < 2. Both represented mild PCOS variants. Hypothalamic disturbances would have been associated with lower LH values and lower testosterone levels. Their acne was also supportive of PCOS. It is possible that they could have represented centrally mediated PCOS.

Case 65

A 27-year-old patient was referred because of irregular menses. Her menarche occurred at age 12 years, followed by menses only one or two times per year, each episode lasting for 21–30 days. At the age of 16 years, she took oral contraceptives for 1 year but discontinued due to poor tolerance. Her past medical history was significant for non-insulin-dependent diabetes mellitus which was diagnosed 4 years prior to her visit and poorly controlled by oral agents. Her family history was positive for diabetes and hypertension. An endometrial biopsy performed by the referring physician showed hyperplasia with mild atypia.

Examination
The patient was an obese African-American female weighing 254 lb (115 kg). Her blood pressure was 130/88 mmHg. She had acanthosis nigricans, was not hirsute and had no galactorrhea. Pelvic examination revealed estrogenic cervical mucus, a normal uterus and no adnexal enlargement.

Laboratory Tests
Thyroid function tests were normal. LH was 3.5 IU/L, FSH was 3.9 IU/L, testosterone was 42 ng/dL, DHEA-S was 254 μg/dL and prolactin was 8 ng/dL.

Follow-up
The patient was treated with medroxyprogesterone acetate, 20 mg daily for 10 days per month for 3 months. The endometrial biopsy was repeated and no atypical hyperplasia was identified. She was subsequently treated with an oral contraceptive of low androgenicity.

Case 66

A 25-year-old patient was referred because of irregular menses, acne and hormone imbalance. Her menarche had occurred at age 12 years, and her menses had always been irregular, occurring every 1 to 4 months. She had had acne since being a teenager, and had also noticed increasing hair growth over her body. There was a family history of diabetes, and her mother was also hirsute.

Examination
Her weight was 142 lb (64.5 kg) and her blood pressure was 110/70 mmHg. She was euthyroid and had no goiter. She had moderate acne and was hirsute over her abdomen, perineum and face. She had acanthosis nigricans over her neck and axillae (Plate 3.2). Pelvic examination revealed a prominent clitoris but was otherwise normal.

Laboratory Tests
TSH was 0.7 μIU/mL, prolactin was 14.2 ng/mL, DHEA-S was 119 μg/dL and testosterone was 118 ng/dL.

Case 67

A 19-year-old patient was referred because of irregular menses and hirsutism. Her menarche occurred at age 12 years, but she had never been regular and would have menses up to 3.5 months apart. She had been hirsute since puberty and also had acne, for which she was taking an antibiotic. There was no history of galactorrhea, weight loss or excessive exercise.

Examination
Her weight was 107 lb (49 kg) and her blood pressure was 110/70 mmHg. She was clinically euthyroid and had no goiter. There was no galactorrhea, but she was moderately hirsute over her face, abdomen and perineum. Pelvic examination was normal.

Laboratory Tests
Her testosterone was 87 ng/dL, DHEA-S was 310 μg/dL, LH was 18.8 IU/L, FSH was 5.2 IU/L and prolactin was 19.4 ng/mL. The results of repeat tests on a subsequent occasion were as follows: testosterone, 40.3 ng/dL; DHEA-S, 340 μg/dL.

Follow-up
She was treated with prednisone, 5 mg at night and 2.5 mg in the morning. Her repeat testosterone and DHEA-S values were 32.4 ng/dL and 200 μg/dL, respectively. Her menses did not normalize.

Discussion of Cases 65–67

In Case 65, the insulin resistance and the inability of the pancreas to respond adequately had precipitated overt diabetes mellitus. In addition, this patient had atypical endometrial hyperplasia, a precursor of endometrial cancer. Case 66 is a typical case of insulin resistance and PCOS exhibiting irregular menses dating from the menarche, as well as acne and hirsutism. Case 67 had a history and physical examination typical of PCOS but was not overweight. Her tests were reflective of predominantly adrenal hyperandrogenism. An ACTH stimulation test could have determined whether she had late-onset congenital adrenal hyperplasia (CAH). During this test, she would have exhibited either a high baseline 17-hydroxyprogestone level (> 200 ng/dL, but only valid during the follicular phase of a cycle) or, more importantly, an exaggerated response to ACTH (nomograms available for interpretation) if she carried this diagnosis. Late onset CAH is an infrequent diagnosis amongst hyperandrogenic women.

Adrenal disorders

ADRENAL HYPERANDROGENISM

Case 68

A 22-year-old patient was seen because of increasing hirsutism of a few years' duration. Her menarche had occurred at age 12 years, and she had had regular monthly cycles until 2 years prior to her visit. In the 2 years preceding her visit her menses had occurred every 3–8 weeks. Her weight had also increased by 35 lb (16 kg) since the age of 15 years.

Examination
Her weight was 175 lb (79.5 kg) and her blood pressure was 122/88 mmHg. She was moderately hirsute over her face, abdomen, hands, feet and perineum. There was no acne, galactorrhea or features of Cushing's syndrome. She also had a prominent clitoris.

Laboratory Tests
Tests performed prior to the patient's visit had revealed testosterone levels of 78 ng/dL, DHEA-S of 918 µg/dL, normal thyroid function and a prolactin level of 9.6 ng/mL. In view of the extremely high DHEA-S value, a 5-day low-dose (2 mg/day) dexamethasone suppression test had been performed, during which the DHEA-S level was suppressed to 115 µg/dL. In addition, an ACTH stimulation test had been performed, during which 250 µg of synthetic ACTH (Cortrosyn) were administered and samples were collected over 1 hour. The baseline 17-hydroxyprogesterone level was 0.89 ng/mL, increasing to 1.9 ng/mL 1 hour post stimulation. The 1-hour 17-hydroxypregnenolone level was 12 ng/mL, giving her a 17-hydroxypregnenolone to 17-hydroxyprogesterone ratio of 6.3 at 1 hour after ACTH stimulation. Serum cortisol on dexamethasone treatment was found to be 2 µg/dL, ruling out Cushing's syndrome.

Follow-up
The patient was given long-term low-dose dexamethasone (0.125–0.25 mg/day) with normalization of her androgens.

Case 69

A 16-year-old patient was seen because of increasing hirsutism over a few years. Her menarche had occurred at age 10.5 years, and she had never had regular menses, these occurring every 2–4 months.

Examination
Her weight was 115 lb (52 kg) and her blood pressure was 90/52 mmHg. She was moderately hirsute over the face, chest and abdomen. There were no features of Cushing's syndrome.

Laboratory Tests
Testosterone was 50 ng/dL, DHEA-S was 1083 μg/dL, prolactin was 13.6 ng/mL and thyroid function was normal. A low-dose (2 mg/day) dexamethasone suppression test reduced her testosterone level to 8.4 ng/dL and her DHEA-S level to 234 μg/dL. An ACTH stimulation test was performed, using 250 μg of synthetic ACTH (Cortrosyn) injected intravenously. Her 17-hydroxypregnenolone was 17.2 ng/mL at 1 hour, giving her a post-stimulation ratio of 17-hydroxypregnenolone to 17-hydroxyprogesterone of 7.2.

Case 70

A 19-year-old patient was seen because of oligomenorrhea, hirsutism and increasing weight gain. Her menarche occurred at age 15 years. She had had no menses for 1 year and then resumed them every 4–6 months.

Examination
Her weight was 250 lb (113.5 kg) and her blood pressure was 126/72 mmHg. She was moderately hirsute but had no features of Cushing's syndrome.

Laboratory Tests
Testosterone was 71 ng/dL, DHEA-S was 606 μg/dL and prolactin ranged from 29 ng/mL to 72 ng/mL. Thyroid function was normal. LH was 11.9 IU/L and FSH was 5.3 IU/L. Low-dose dexamethasone (2 mg/day) suppression reduced her testosterone level to 20 ng/dL and her DHEA-S level to 103 μg/dL over 2 days. A cortisol level of 0.9 μg/dL at this time ruled out Cushing's syndrome. An ACTH stimulation test was performed using 250 μg of synthetic ACTH (Cortrosyn) given intravenously. The 17-hydroxyprogesterone level rose from 0.58 ng/mL to 1.2 ng/mL over 1 hour, and her 17-hydroxypregnenolone level at 1 hour was 10.6 ng/mL, giving a 17-hydroxypregnenolone to 17-hydroxyprogesterone ratio of 8.8 at 1 hour post stimulation.

CONGENITAL ADRENAL HYPERPLASIA

Case 71

A 16-year-old patient was seen because of secondary amenorrhea. At the age of 3 months she was noted to have clitoromegaly, but no action was taken. At the age of 5 years, she had a tonsillectomy and her recovery was uneventful except for a febrile episode post-operatively. At the age of 6 years, she had developed some pubic hairs, her clitoris had continued to enlarge and hormonal tests were performed. She was diagnosed with simple virilizing 21-hydroxylase deficiency and was treated with prednisone initially, but this was subsequently switched to hydrocortisone because of its shorter duration of action (and possibly less inhibitory effect on growth). Despite an advanced bone age, she grew to a final height of 5 feet 1 inch (155 cm). She had her first period at the age of 14 years, but her menses were erratic, and at the time of her visit she had been amenorrheic for 9 months. She was taking hydrocortisone, 10 mg in the morning, 7.5 mg at noon and 7.5 mg in the evening. Resection of the clitoris had been performed at the age of 8 years.

Examination
Her weight was 116 lb (53 kg) and her height was 5 feet 1 inch (155 cm). She was mildly hirsute, had well-developed breasts, and a limited pelvic examination was normal.

Laboratory Tests
The following tests were obtained at 8 a.m.: cortisol, 3 µg/dL (low); ACTH, 41 pg/mL (normal range 0–70 pg/mL); 17-hydroxyprogesterone, 39.7 ng/mL (normal follicular phase 0.15–0.7); testosterone, 62 ng/dL; dehydroepiandrosterone, 33 µg/dL; prolactin, 7.7 ng/mL; LH, 1.1 IU/L; FSH, 4.9 IU/L.

Follow-up
She was switched to dexamethasone, 0.25 mg twice daily. Her testosterone level fell to below the limit of detection, and her 17-hydroxyprogesterone level fell to 1.16 ng/mL. On this regimen, her plasma renin activity was determined. It was found to be elevated and fludrocortisone was added to her treatment regimen.

Case 72

A 16-year-old patient was referred for continuing management of 21-hydroxylase deficiency congenital adrenal hyperplasia. The diagnosis had been made at the age of 2 years, following the discovery of pubic hair. She was treated initially with hydrocortisone and after the age of 14 years with prednisone and fludrocortisone. Her 17-hydroxyprogesterone level had been elevated and out of control twice, and the doses of her medications were increased. Her current medication consisted of prednisone, 5 mg twice daily, and fludrocortisone, 0.15 mg daily. She had clitoral reduction surgery at the age of 4 years. Her bone age had remained close to her chronological age. She started breast development at the age of 11.5 years and had her first period at the age of 14 years. Her menses were regular, and there was no family history of congenital adrenal hyperplasia.

Examination
Her height was 4 feet 11 inches (150 cm); her father was 5 feet 6 inches (168 cm) tall and her mother was 5 feet 0 inches (152 cm) tall. She was clinically euthyroid and had no goiter. There was mild excess abdominal hair. Her breasts were well developed and the external genitalia were normal. She did not consent to pelvic examination.

Laboratory Tests
Tests were performed in the follicular phase of her cycle. Her electrolytes were normal. Her 17-hydroxyprogesterone level was 0.42 ng/mL (normal follicular phase 0.15–0.7 ng/mL) and androstenedione was 26 ng/dL (normal range 85–275 ng/dL). Her plasma renin activity was 92 ng/dL/hour (normal upright range is 70–330 ng/dL/hour).

Discussion of Cases 68–72

Cases 68–70 had extremely high DHEA-S concentrations. Such high levels reflect adrenal hypersecretion, and all of them responded to ACTH suppression using dexamethasone. It has been suggested that a partial deficiency of 3β-hydroxy-dehydrogenase exists in some of these patients, and the test recommended for determining such deficiency is again an ACTH stimulation test. A high ratio of 17-hydroxypregnenolone to 17-hydroxyprogesterone (> 8) is said to be confirmatory. However, another school of thought is that in these patients the adrenal 17α-hydroxylase enzyme system has exaggerated function. Case 70 also had mild to moderate hyperprolactinemia, which is sometimes seen in PCOS–chronic anovulation and may reflect the hyperestrogenic state of these patients (estrogens prime the lactotroph, leading to increased prolactin concentrations, and this is presumed to explain the hyperprolactinemia of pregnancy as well).

Cases 71 and 72 were two patients with congenital adrenal hyperplasia (CAH) due to 21-hydroxylase deficiency, diagnosed in early childhood. The adrenal steroidogenic pathway is shown in Figure 4.1. Neither of them had been salt-losing, and both had presented with early virilization. The diagnosis of 21-hydroxylase deficiency, the commonest form of CAH, inherited in autosomal-recessive fashion (with genetic linkage to the human leukocyte antigen (HLA) system) is made by an ACTH stimulation test, during which a very exaggerated response to ACTH is observed (nomograms available for diagnosis). The treatment consists of suppression of ACTH with glucocorticoids, but it may be difficult to find the appropriate dose because too high a dose will suppress growth, while too low a dose will lead to inadequate androgen suppression. Mineralocorticoid treatment using fludrocortisone is often necessary in these patients in order to reduce further ACTH stimulation that results from inadequate aldosterone production. Uncontrolled CAH (as in Case 71 at presentation at the age of 16 years) is often associated with chronic anovulation and a picture of PCOS. Although the diagnosis of Cases 71 and 72 was CAH, patients may present *de novo* with hirsutism, acne and chronic anovulation post-pubertally, and are then said to have 'late-onset' CAH. This diagnosis can be made by means of an ACTH stimulation test. Synthetic ACTH (250 μg) is administered intravenously and 17-hydroxyprogesterone is determined at baseline and at 30 and 60 minutes. An exaggerated response is characteristic of CAH. In most studies, late-onset CAH represents only a small proportion of patients with PCOS (5% or less).

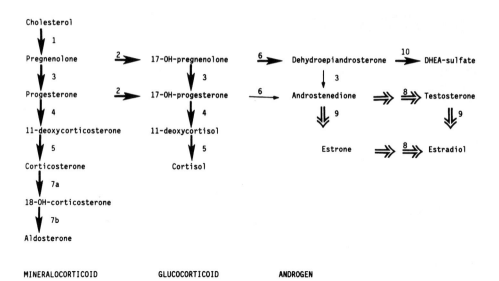

Figure 4.1 Adrenal steroidogenic pathways of mineralocorticoid, glucocorticoid and androgen synthesis. Major pathways are indicated by thick arrows and minor ones are denoted by thin arrows. Extra-adrenal conversion of sex steroids is denoted by double arrows. Numbers indicate enzymatic steps as follows: 1, 20α-hydroxylase, 22-hydroxylase, 20–22 desmolase; 2, 17α-hydroxylase; 3, 3β-hydroxysteroid dehydrogenase, 5–4 isomerase; 4, 21-hydroxylase; 5, 11β-hydroxylase; 6, C17–20 lyase; 7a, 18-hydroxylase; 7b, 18-dehydrogenase; 8, 17β-hydroxysteroid dehydrogenase; 9, aromatase; 10, sulfatase.

5

Thyroid disorders

Case 73

A 25-year-old patient presented with a history of irregular menses. Her menarche occurred at age 11 years with the establishment of regular menses within 4 months. She took oral contraceptives from the age of 19 years and discontinued them 4 months prior to her visit. During these 4 months her menses were irregular and more prolonged. She had gained 4 lb (2 kg) in weight and had noticed slight acne since discontinuing the oral contraceptives.

Examination
Her weight was 133 lb (60 kg) and her blood pressure was 108/64 mmHg. She was clinically euthyroid and her thyroid was just palpable. There was no galactorrhea and minimal excess hair, and pelvic examination was normal.

Laboratory Tests
T_4 was 9.1 µg/dL, T_3 resin uptake was 28% and TSH was 17.4 µIU/mL. Her anti-microsomal antibody was strongly positive and the antithyroglobulin antibody was negative. Her prolactin level was 7.2 ng/mL, DHEA-S was 149 µg/dL and testosterone was 24 ng/dL.

Discussion of Case 73

This patient had established normal menses at menarche and continued to show a normal pattern until the onset of birth control pill therapy. After discontinuing the pill, she had irregular, more prolonged menses and she gained a small amount of weight. Evaluation revealed hypothyroidism of autoimmune etiology (see Glossary of Common Tests on p. 213). Hypothyroidism can be associated with menstrual dysfunction, and several mechanisms may play a role. In primary hypothyroidism, as thyrotropin-releasing hormone (TRH) levels are elevated, prolactin is also commonly elevated, as TRH stimulates the production and release of both TSH and prolactin. It is for this reason that galactorrhea also sometimes occurs in patients with primary hypothyroidism. In addition, alteration of the metabolism of androgens and estrogens and changes in sex-hormone-binding globulin may also lead to a state of chronic anovulation not dissimilar to that seen in polycystic ovary syndrome. Finally, menstrual flow is often described as heavier and more prolonged in hypothyroidism and as scantier in hyperthyroidism.

PREGNANCY-RELATED DISORDERS

Case 74

A 21-year-old patient who was 12.5 weeks pregnant was referred because of abnormal thyroid function tests in the setting of hyperemesis gravidarum. This was her second pregnancy, her first having occurred at the age of 20 years; that pregnancy had been terminated at 6 weeks and she had been asymptomatic. Seven weeks into her current pregnancy, she developed severe nausea and vomiting, and by the time she attended, she had lost 13 lb (6 kg) in weight. Thyroid function tests performed at 7 weeks had shown a suppressed TSH with a normal free thyroxine index and T_3. By 9 weeks, with the progression of her symptoms, her T_4 was 19.8 μg/dL, T_3 resin uptake was 29%, the free thyroxine index was 5.7 and TSH was < 0.03 μIU/mL. She gave no history of thyroid disease and was otherwise asymptomatic, but her mother had Graves' disease and had been treated with radioactive iodine. After a brief period of hospitalization, the patient had been treated with promethazine and metoclopramide and was better.

Examination
Her weight was 116 lb (53 kg), her blood pressure was 100/60 mmHg and her pulse was regular at 88 beats/minute. She was clinically euthyroid and had no goiter. There was no tremor, her skin temperature was normal and she had no ocular abnormalities.

Laboratory Tests
Tests performed at 12.5 weeks' gestation were as follows. T_4 was 13.8 μg/dL, T_3 resin uptake was 23%, free thyroxine index was 3.2 and TSH was 0.8 μIU/L (normal). Free thyroxine was 1.04 ng/dL (normal range 0.7–2.0 ng/dL), free T_3 was 2.5 pg/mL (normal range 2.3–4.2 pg/mL), antithyroid antibodies were negative and an erythrocyte zinc determination was within the normal range.

Case 75

A 33-year-old patient was referred for evaluation of abnormal thyroid function tests. She had complained of palpitations, tremor and tiredness for a few months, as well as slight menstrual irregularity. Thyroid function tests performed several weeks prior to her visit had revealed a T_4 of 12.7 µg/dL, a T_3 resin uptake of 33% and a suppressed TSH of less than 0.3 µIU/mL. Her medical history was otherwise negative. She had recently had an uneventful pregnancy and had delivered approximately 3 months prior to the onset of her symptoms.

Examination
Her weight was 160½ lb (73 kg), her blood pressure was 120/80 mmHg and her pulse was regular at 92 beats/minute. She was slightly sweaty, but examination was otherwise negative. Her thyroid gland was of upper normal size and without tenderness.

Laboratory Tests
T_4 was 8.3 µg/dL, T_3 resin uptake was 30% and TSH was less than 0.3 µIU/mL. Her antimicrosomal (thyroid peroxidase) antibodies were negative but her anti-thyroglobulin antibodies were strongly positive. Radionucleotide thyroid scanning showed extremely poor uptake with ^{123}I uptake of 2% at 4 hours and 1% at 24 hours (see Glossary of Common Tests on p. 213).

Case 76

A 34-year-old patient was referred because of hyperthyroidism. She was 18 weeks pregnant, and prior to this pregnancy, she had been evaluated by an endocrinologist for ovulatory dysfunction and had serum thyrotropin levels measured, which were found to be normal. At 9 weeks' gestation she developed extreme nausea and vomiting. Thyroid function tests were repeated at this time, and her TSH was suppressed at < 0.1 μIU/mL and she had a free thyroxine level of 2.12 ng/dL (normal range 0.8–2.0 ng/dL). She was referred for high-risk obstetrical care, and a repeat TSH measurement at approximately 15 weeks' pregnancy was < 0.03 μIU/mL. By 18 weeks' gestation, although her symptoms were abating, it was noted that she had only gained 3.5 lb (1.6 kg in weight).

Examination
The patient was clinically euthyroid with a regular pulse rate of 76 beats/minute. She had no thyroid enlargement, no tremor and no evidence of thyroid eye disease.

Laboratory Tests
Free thyroxine was 0.8 ng/dL, free tri-iodothyronine was 370 pg/dL (normal range 250–550 pg/dL), TSH was 0.52 μIU/mL (normal range 0.4–5.5 μIU/mL) and antithyroid antibodies were negative.

Case 77

A 32-year-old patient was referred with hyperthyroidism. She presented with tachycardia, increased appetite and tremors. Thyroid function tests showed excessive thyroid hormones and a 24-hour iodine uptake study demonstrated an elevated uptake of 51%. Shortly after these tests, pregnancy was diagnosed and the patient started on propylthiouracil (PTU), 300 mg daily. Despite 9 weeks of such treatment, her tri-iodothyronine level was significantly elevated at 389 ng/dL, and her TSH level was suppressed. Her dose of PTU was increased to 600 mg daily a few days prior to her visit. She was also given propranolol, 40 mg twice daily. There was a strong family history of hypothyroidism.

Examination

On examination, the patient was warm and sweaty and had mild proptosis. Her pulse rate was 76 beats/minute. She had a diffuse 40-gram goiter.

Case 78

A 27-year-old patient was referred for evaluation and management of thyroid dysfunction. Six months after a normal delivery following an uneventful pregnancy, she experienced tiredness, weakness and drowsiness. Tests revealed a T_4 of 3.8 µg/dL, a low free thyroxine index and a TSH of 53 µIU/mL. There was no past history of thyroid disease or surgery.

Examination
Although she was not overtly hypothyroid, she had a 35-gram firm diffuse goiter.

Laboratory Tests
Antithyroid antibodies were negative 2 months after the onset of her symptoms and after the initiation of thyroid hormone replacement.

Follow-up
She was treated with appropriate doses of thyroxine for 18 months, during which time she had another uneventful pregnancy. Six months after this delivery, she had a barely palpable thyroid. Thyroxine therapy was discontinued and the patient was observed closely. Two months later, her T_4 was 8.7 µg/dL, T_3 resin uptake was 26%, free thyroxine index was 2.3 and TSH was 3 µIU/mL (normal range 0.32–5 µIU/mL). She remained off thyroxine replacement therapy. Repeat tests 8 months after cessation of replacement therapy were as follows: T_4, 3.5 µg/dL; T_3 resin uptake, 28%; free thyroxine index, 1.0 (low); TSH, 28 µIU/mL. Thyroxine therapy was restarted.

Case 79

A 24-year-old patient was referred for evaluation of thyroid dysfunction. She had been in good health, had delivered her second child 4 months prior to her visit, and all had been well until 4 weeks prior to her visit. At this time, she complained of palpitations, difficulty in breathing and a significant weight loss. There was a family history of thyroid disease. Laboratory tests by her referring physician had shown a T_4 of 18.2 μg/dL, a T_3 resin uptake of 33%, a free thyroxine index of 6 (normal range 1–4) and a suppressed TSH of < 0.3 μIU/mL.

Examination
She was slightly sweaty, her pulse rate was 80 beats/minute, and her thyroid was just palpable.

Laboratory Tests
Repeat thyroid function tests were as follows: T_4 13 μg/dL; T_3 resin uptake, 31%; free thyroxine index, 4.0; TSH, < 0.03 μIU/mL. Antimicrosomal antibodies were strongly positive. ^{123}I uptake revealed a very suppressed uptake of 1.7% and 1.2% at 4 and 24 hours, respectively.

Follow-up
Her symptoms improved without treatment. Three weeks after her initial visit, her T_4 was 5.8 μg/dL, T_3 resin uptake was 28%, free thyroxine index was 1.6, and TSH was 0.13 μIU/mL (normal range 0.32–5 μIU/mL). Eight weeks after her initial visit, her T_4 was 4.6 μg/dL (normal range 4.5–12.5 μg/dL), T_3 resin uptake was 29%, free thyroxine index was 1.3 and TSH was 24.4 μIU/mL.

Discussion of Cases 74–79

Figures 5.1 and 5.2 outline the evaluation and management of thyrotoxicosis in pregnancy (Figure 5.1) and postpartum (Figure 5.2). Case 77 demonstrates the combination of two common diagnoses, namely Graves' disease and pregnancy. Graves' disease is an autoimmune thyroid disease. The autoimmune process involves the production of thyroid-stimulating immunoglobulins which activate the thyroid TSH receptor, leading to overproduction of the hormones thyroxine (T_4) and tri-iodothyronine (T_3). The gland is usually diffusely enlarged, as in this case, the 24-hour iodine uptake is usually elevated, and there may be a family history of thyroid disease. In this patient, the diagnosis was established at the same time as that of pregnancy. There are three modalities of treatment for hyperthyroidism, namely antithyroid medications, partial thyroidectomy and radioactive iodine therapy. Clearly radioactive iodine is contraindicated in pregnancy, and antithyroid medications have long been used to treat hyperthyroidism in this circumstance. The drug of choice is propylthiouracil (PTU) rather than methimazole, which has been associated with a scalp defect known as cutis aplasia (methimazole is similar to carbimazole, which is available in Europe and Canada). Although PTU readily crosses the placenta and may cause a fetal goiter, if given in excess dosage it has no other significant fetal effects, and its use in pregnancy is safe. As with non-pregnant patients, there is a possibility of side-effects such as a maculopapular rash (c. 5%) or agranulocytosis, which is rare (1% of cases) but potentially very serious. Due to its ability to cross the placenta, and because women generally tolerate a mild state of hyperthyroidism well in pregnancy, it is recommended that large doses should not be used. However, as illustrated by this case, it is important to control overt hyperthyroidism adequately, and doses of 600 mg or so can be used in selected pregnant women, provided that the patient is monitored closely and the dose reduced as soon as she approaches the euthyroid state. As in non-pregnant patients, propranolol may also be used in pregnancy to reduce sympathetic overactivity, although this is done with a degree of reluctance by some obstetricians because of the reputed association with growth retardation. It may be stopped as soon as the euthyroid state is achieved.

Significantly hyperthyroid patients have an increased risk of fetal demise, premature delivery, premature closure of scalp growth plates and low birth weight. After achieving a euthyroid state, the dose of PTU can be reduced every few weeks and the lowest dose maintained so long as euthyroidism is maintained. As pregnancy represents a state of relative immune tolerance, the disease may remit spontaneously, and it has therefore been suggested that PTU therapy can often be discontinued in the third trimester. However, it is important to remember that in the postpartum period there is often relapse (or initial appearance) of immunologically mediated conditions, such as Graves' disease. If PTU is discontinued, such patients should be closely observed during the year following delivery.

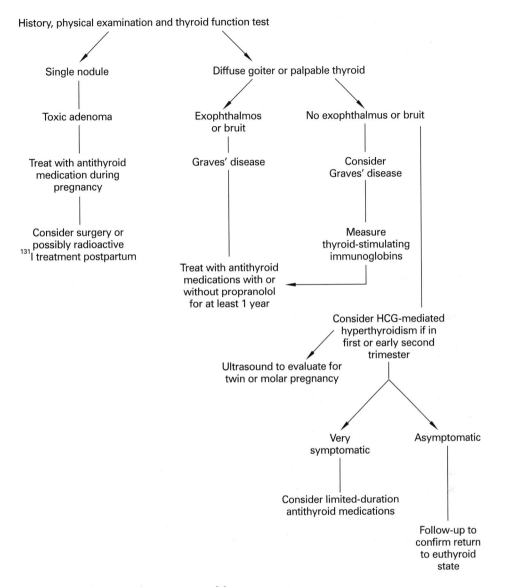

Figure 5.1 Evaluation and management of thyrotoxicosis in pregnancy.

If surgical therapy becomes necessary (e.g. because of side-effects with PTU) it should preferably be performed in the second trimester in a patient whose over-activity has been blocked by PTU, propranolol and also iodine to reduce the vascularity of the gland. It should be remembered that iodine readily crosses the placenta, and that in large, prolonged doses it may lead to fetal goiter and hypothyroidism.

Neonatal thyrotoxicosis may rarely occur in an infant born to a mother with Graves' disease, even if her Graves' disease has been treated. Approximately one in 70 women with a history of Graves' disease will have a clinically affected infant.

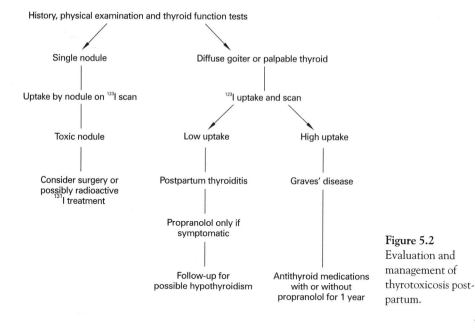

History, physical examination and thyroid function tests

Single nodule

Diffuse goiter or palpable thyroid

Uptake by nodule on ^{123}I scan

^{123}I uptake and scan

Toxic nodule

Low uptake

High uptake

Consider surgery or possibly radioactive ^{131}I treatment

Postpartum thyroiditis

Graves' disease

Propranolol only if symptomatic

Follow-up for possible hypothyroidism

Antithyroid medications with or without propranolol for 1 year

Figure 5.2 Evaluation and management of thyrotoxicosis postpartum.

Such an infant has an enlarged thyroid, ocular signs such as prominence and stare, may be small for his or her gestational age, and is agitated, hyperkinetic and possibly hyperthermic. In mothers with Graves' disease treated in pregnancy, this may be manifested in the infant clinically and biochemically within a few days of delivery when the effect of the transplacentally transferred PTU has worn off. In these circumstances, neonatal thyrotoxicosis is due to transplacental crossing of maternally derived thyroid-stimulating immunoglobulins (TSH receptor-stimulating antibodies). Assays for these antibodies are available and will confirm the cause of the neonatal thyrotoxicosis. These immunoglobulins disappear within 3 to 6 months, but the infant may require treatment with PTU, propranolol and iodide until resolution and disappearance of the immunoglobulins.

Case 75 is a 33-year-old patient who developed symptoms of hyperthyroidism within a few months postpartum, and whose initial thyroid function test results are consistent with thyrotoxicosis. At the time of her visit, her thyroid was of upper-normal size and not tender. Repeat thyroid function tests showed some recovery in that her previously elevated T_4 level was now normal. Antithyroid antibodies were positive and radionucleotide uptake showed extremely poor uptake. Diminished iodine uptake together with excess thyroid hormone are the hallmarks of thyroiditis. Subacute (de Quervain's) thyroiditis is viral, usually affecting subjects in the setting of an upper respiratory infection. The gland is enlarged, painful and tender, and T_4 and T_3 levels may be elevated because of outpouring of hormones from an inflamed gland, which does not concentrate iodine.

The patient described here had no pain or tenderness. There is a second form of thyroiditis called *painless thyroiditis*, which almost always affects women, usually a few months postpartum. It is an autoimmune disease (hence the positive antibodies, usually antimicrosomal or antithyroid peroxidase antibodies) belonging to the same group of disorders exemplified by Graves' disease and Hashimoto's thyroiditis (with or without hypothyroidism). It manifests postpartum because this is the time when autoimmune diseases may make their initial appearance. The gland is inflamed (hence the low iodine uptake), and outpouring of thyroid hormone leads to the manifestations of hyperthyroidism. It is a self-limiting disease, the symptoms and hyperthyroidism resolving within a few weeks, as in this case. Antithyroid medications such as PTU are not indicated, but propranolol may be used to reduce sympathetic overactivity. During recovery, transient hypothyroidism may also occur, and a certain proportion of these patients (approximately 25%) may subsequently become permanently hypothyroid, so long-term follow-up is desirable. Case 79 also had painless thyroiditis. She became hypothyroid during recovery. In most cases this is a transient phenomenon although, as indicated above, permanent hypothyroidism may occur subsequently.

Case 78 also represents autoimmune disease occurring postpartum. This patient was completely well during and in the few months following her delivery. Approximately 6 months postpartum she became symptomatic and was found to be hypothyroid with a small firm goiter. She did not manifest any hyperthyroid phase. Because of the postpartum nature of her problem and the transient occurrence of autoimmune diseases at this time, thyroxine therapy was discontinued after her following pregnancy. Although she was initially euthyroid when off therapy, she subsequently lapsed into hypothyroidism, confirming the need for lifelong treatment with thyroxine in her case.

Case 76 was documented to be biochemically euthyroid prior to a pregnancy, but symptoms of nausea, vomiting and inadequate weight gain led to the discovery of hyperthyroidism at 9 weeks' gestation. By the time she was seen by an endocrinologist at 18 weeks' gestation, her symptoms had abated and she was clinically and biochemically euthyroid. This patient, with manifestations of hyperthyroidism in the first and early second trimester that later resolved, almost certainly has human chorionic gonadotropin (HCG) mediated hyperthyroidism with associated hyperemesis gravidarum. HCG is a weak thyroid-stimulating hormone that occupies the TSH receptor. Different HCG molecules with different carbohydrate and sialic acid components have differing abilities to activate the TSH receptor and induce hyperthyroidism. In addition, a mutant TSH receptor may be present that is more responsive to HCG (Rodien, P., Bremont, C., Sanson, M.-L. R. et al. 1998: Familial gestational hyperthyroidism caused by a mutant thyrotropin receptor hypersensitive to HCG. New England Journal of Medicine 339, 1823). Since HCG levels are highest at approximately 10 weeks' gestation, this is when the patient is likely to be symptomatic, with her symptoms abating during the second trimester. These patients have no signs of autoimmune disease and no goiter, and in contrast to Graves' disease, which often improves in pregnancy, they present for the first time with symptoms in pregnancy. As it is a self-resolving process, treatment is conservative and consists of hydration, intravenous nutrition or hyperalimentation as necessary. There may be a role for short-term antithyroid hormone therapy, but this is likely to be limited by nausea and vomiting, and there is little literature on this issue.

Case 74 also presented with hyperemesis and weight loss in early pregnancy. She became progressively more hyperthyroid biochemically, but improved after 12 weeks' gestation. The history is complicated by a family history of Graves' disease (her mother had it). Tests performed at 12.5 weeks show attainment of euthyroid status, and she had no goiter or ocular manifestations of Graves' disease. Her antithyroid antibodies were negative. Again, despite the family history, it is likely that this patient had HCG-mediated hyperthyroidism which resolved by the second trimester. Her normal erythrocyte zinc level was consistent with the diagnosis, as it is said to be depleted in patients with Graves' disease.

Case 80

A 32-year-old patient was referred for management of hypothyroidism in pregnancy. A few years prior to her visit, she had received radioactive iodine for Graves' disease and had subsequently become hypothyroid. She was placed on L-thyroxine, 0.1 mg, and had documented normal thyroid function tests a few months before becoming pregnant. Towards the end of her first trimester she complained of tiredness and sluggishness. Repeat thyroid function tests found an elevated TSH of 11 μIU/mL. Her dose of L-thyroxine was increased to 0.112 mg.

Examination
The patient was clinically euthyroid and had no goiter.

Follow-up
She eventually required approximately 0.2 mg of L-thyroxine to achieve a normal TSH.

Discussion of Case 80

Current management of primary hypothyroidism dictates that a dose of thyroxine sufficient to keep the TSH within the normal range should be administered. Overdosage is undesirable because of its potential for causing bone loss and possible cardiac effects. The requirements for thyroxine may increase during pregnancy as illustrated in Case 80. At least two factors play a role in this increased requirement. First, the fetal requirement may place demands on the maternal thyroid, which the mother cannot meet because of thyroid destruction. Secondly, iron and prenatal vitamins containing iron may interfere with thyroxine absorption. Patients should be advised to take their thyroxine many hours apart from their iron and vitamins, and the dosage should be increased appropriately to bring the elevated TSH level back down to within the normal range.

Menopause

6

BREAST CANCER/BONE LOSS

Case 81

A 42-year-old patient was referred for advice on menopausal status and its management. Eighteen months prior to her visit she had had bilateral mastectomies for breast cancer. This was followed by seven courses of chemotherapy which rendered her menopausal, and she had had some hot flashes. She did not smoke or drink, and there was no family history of osteoporosis. Her only medications were 1000 mg calcium per day and a multivitamin.

Examination
She weighed 171 lb (78 kg) and her height was 6 feet 1 inch (185 cm). She was clinically euthyroid and had no goiter. Apart from the mastectomies, examination was negative. Pelvic examination revealed mild vaginal mucosal atrophy.

Laboratory Tests
Thyroid function tests were normal. A recent bone mineral density study had not shown her to be at risk of fracture. A repeat examination 9 months later showed a 3.5% decrease in the bone mineral density of the lateral lumbar spine, and a 2–5% decrease in the bone mineral density of her left hip.

Follow-up
Treatment options were discussed and the patient was started on alendronate, a bisphosphonate.

Case 82

A 42-year-old patient attended to discuss issues pertaining to the menopause. Her menarche occurred the age of 13 years, and she had regular cycles. During the last few months she had experienced some hot flashes and a few night sweats. She had no significant past illnesses, but review of her family history revealed a strong history of breast cancer. Her mother had developed the disease at the age of 34 years, her grandmother at the age of 56 years, and her maternal aunt at the age of 40 years. There was no family history of osteoporosis, heart disease or ovarian cancer.

Examination
Breast, general and pelvic examinations were normal.

Laboratory Tests
Her mammogram was normal.

Case 83

A 51-year-old Caucasian woman presented to obtain advice on prevention of osteoporosis. She had a normal reproductive history and had had two pregnancies. At the age of 48 years, a hysterectomy and bilateral oophorectomy had been performed for benign disease. She was promptly treated with estrogen replacement in standard dosage. Just prior to her visit, multifocal lobular carcinoma *in situ* of the breast had been diagnosed, and she had bilateral mastectomies performed. She came off estrogen treatment at this time. Although she was told that there was little likelihood of recurrence, based on the initial histology, the patient was reluctant to take estrogens. Her grandmother had fractured a hip at the age of 62 years following a fall.

Examination
Her weight was 111 lb (50 kg). She was clinically euthyroid and, apart from mastectomy scars, her general physical examination was unremarkable.

Laboratory Tests
Bone mineral density studies were performed both at the time of her visit and 8 months later. During these 8 months she sustained approximately 4% bone loss, on the basis of measurements over her hip and spine.

Follow-up
She was treated with subcutaneous calcitonin, 50 IU on alternate days. Repeat bone density measurements using the same machine over 5 years of follow-up showed bone loss of approximately 2% during this time period. Subsequently, the patient decided to take estrogen therapy because of her concerns about heart disease and memory loss. After 2.5 years of estrogen plus calcitonin therapy, a gain of bone of approximately 4% (average of hip and spine) was recorded.

Case 84

A 40-year-old patient was referred for routine evaluation and to discuss issues relating to the menopause. Her menarche occurred at age 13 years, and she had irregular menses and was told that she had polycystic ovary syndrome. At the age of 19 years, she was diagnosed with invasive breast cancer and had undergone a bilateral mastectomy. Her tumor was estrogen-receptor-positive. Her menses had become more regular with time. She was a non-smoker, and her mother had sustained an ulnar fracture following a fall at the age of 68 years and had lost some height. Her paternal grandmother had had breast cancer and her great aunt had had ovarian cancer.

Examination
She weighed 144 lb (65 kg) and was moderately hirsute and clinically euthyroid. Pelvic examination was unremarkable.

Laboratory Tests
Her testosterone level was 30 ng/dL and her DHEA-S level was 125 μg/dL.

Discussion of Cases 81–84

Patients with breast cancer who are perimenopausal or in early menopause pose a special therapeutic problem, especially with regard to bone loss progressing to osteoporosis. Osteoporosis is a systemic skeletal disease characterized by low bone mass and microarchitectural deterioration of bone tissue leading to a susceptibility to fracture. The fractures associated with osteoporosis are related to a multifactorial pathophysiology that incorporates bone mass, falls, postural reflexes, body habitus and age. For women in their early menopausal years, estrogen deficiency is the dominant influence on bone loss. Dual X-ray absorptiometry (DXA) scans measure bone mineral density (BMD) in grams per square centimeter, and are useful tools for monitoring bone density of patients due to the low radiation exposure. The precision is sufficient to allow long-term monitoring. Several clinical studies have demonstrated that low BMD values are associated with an increased risk of fracture. Based on clinical associations between BMD and fracture risk, the World Health Organization has outlined parameters for osteoporosis diagnosis. A BMD between 1 and 2.5 standard deviations (SD) *below a young normal reference group* is said to define *osteopenia*. If the BMD is equal to or less than 2.5 SD below young normal BMD levels, *osteoporosis* is diagnosed. A normal BMD is defined as a value within one SD of young normal adults. Comparison of an individual's BMD at any given site with that of young normal adults defines the t-score. Thus a person with a t-score of −1.25 SD at the lumbar spine is said to have osteopenia of the lumbar spine. Most BMD reports also record a z-score, which compares that individual's BMD with the BMD levels of individuals of the same age and sex. Risk factors for osteoporosis include family history, ethnicity (there is higher risk among East Asians compared to Caucasians and African-Americans), smoking, low body weight and thin frame, medications such as glucocorticoids, excess thyroid hormones, heparin, anticonvulsants and a hypogonadal state.

Table 6.1 shows an example of a BMD report.

Table 6.1 Bone mineral density: example of a report

	BMD (g/cm^2)	Peak bone mass		Age/sex-matched	
		t-score	%	z-score	%
Lumbar spine					
Anterior	0.664	−3.48	63	−3.13	66
Lateral	0.575	−2.91	78	−2.14	76
Left hip					
Neck	0.751	−1.44	84	−0.84	90
Trochanter	0.526	−2.18	73	−1.93	75
Intertrochanter	0.776	−2.66	68	−2.42	70
Total	0.678	−2.47	70	−2.20	72
Ward's triangle	0.530	−2.42	67	−1.26	79

Case 81 developed breast cancer and was rendered menopausal by the age of 41 years by the chemotherapy administered postoperatively. She did not smoke, had no other significant risk factors, and bone mineral density studies performed shortly after her cancer treatment had shown no increased fracture risk. However, repeat densitometry performed 9 months later had shown significant loss of bone, despite reasonable calcium and vitamin therapy. This loss of bone is not unexpected in a menopausal patient who is not on estrogen replacement therapy. Because of her breast cancer, this patient was not a suitable candidate for estrogen/progestin replacement, and protection against bone loss related to estrogen deficiency becomes a high priority in these circumstances. Calcium supplementation at 1500 mg/day is recommended, together with vitamin D, 400–800 IU daily, but this is not sufficient to ward off bone loss. Lack of estrogen allows accelerated bone resorption, and normal bone formation is unable to keep up with the losses. Agents that inhibit osteoclastic bone resorption are recommended, and currently two classes of medications are approved for the treatment of osteoporosis. The first is calcitonin, a hormone normally produce by the C-cells of the thyroid. Calcitonin's effect is exerted on bone osteoclasts, inhibiting their action. It is available both as subcutaneous injections and as a nasal spray, and its side-effects consist mainly of flushing. The second class of agents consists of the bisphosphonates – currently alendronate is approved for this purpose, and others are pending approval (e.g. risedronate). Bisphosphonates are absorbed from the gastrointestinal tract, taken up by bone tissue and inhibit bone resorption. For the prevention of osteoporosis, they are administered orally. The major side-effects of alendronate are gastrointestinal. A third class of agents with a long history of use for osteoporosis treatment and fracture prevention consists of fluoride. This drug is controversial, as although bone density is increased, the bone architecture is structurally defective and abnormal. The formulation of the preparation and the supplementary calcium and vitamin D used may also play important roles in its efficacy. Certain formulations may be approved for osteoporosis in future. Selective estrogen-receptor modulators, such as raloxifene, also reduce bone loss. Although not specifically approved for patients with breast cancer, their lack of action (and probable protective effect) on breasts would suggest their usefulness in patients with breast cancer.

Treatment of hot flashes in women who are unable to take estrogens can also be problematic. Clonidine, acting centrally, has been used with some success, usually in the form of transdermal patches. Bellergal and barbiturates have also been helpful in some patients. Fortunately, these symptoms usually wear off with time.

Case 84 also developed breast cancer premenopausally and had a family history of both breast and ovarian cancer. She did not have chemotherapy, so she was still menstruating. Calcium and vitamin D supplementation was advised, as was surveillance for bone loss. Significant bone loss would warrant pharmacologic intervention as discussed above.

Case 83 had been rendered surgically menopausal at the age of 48 years, but had the benefit of 3 years of estrogen therapy prior to the diagnosis of lobular carcinoma of the breast at age 51 years. Although hormone replacement therapy was not contraindicated in her case, given the *in-situ* nature of her disease and her bilateral mastectomies, she was reluctant to take it any longer. She was thin, and had a family history of hip fracture at age 62 years. Bone mineral density studies performed twice during the year after her cancer treatment showed significant loss of bone. She received subcutaneous calcitonin and over 6 years of follow-up sustained only 2% average bone loss, indicating the efficacy of calcitonin in her case. She subsequently reconsidered estrogen therapy, mainly for its cardioprotective effects and reinitiated it. Raloxifene offers some cardioprotection and would be a suitable alternative.

Case 82 was perimenopausal at the time of her first visit, and she sought advice about future estrogen replacement therapy. She clearly had a very significant family history of breast cancer, with multiple family members involved, several at a very young age. Cancer-screening mammograms are recommended annually in such cases, starting 5 years prior to the age of diagnosis of the youngest case. It is still the subject of debate whether estrogen replacement therapy increases a woman's lifetime risk of breast cancer, but recent studies suggest that there may be a small increase in risk. This patient is already at major risk, which could theoretically be compounded by estrogen treatment. In the current state of knowledge, it may be reasonable to withhold estrogen treatment from this patient at the time of menopause, although the use of genetic markers to identify those at risk may aid in decision-making. Raloxifene may also be an appropriate choice. In the absence of a strong family history, such as that described above, and with only one first-degree family member affected, it is not necessary to withhold estrogen therapy. However, close surveillance both by clinical and self-examination and by annual mammography is mandatory.

Case 85

A 43-year-old patient was referred for management of hormone replacement. Her menarche occurred at age 11 years, and for the most part she had regular cycles until the age of approximately 32 years. At this time she developed a rheumatologic problem and was treated with cyclophosphamide, and she also had her right ovary removed because of benign disease. Within 6 months of these two events she became amenorrheic. Six years later she had a hysterectomy for cervical dysplasia, and post-operatively she received conjugated equine estrogens (CEE), 1.25 mg, for 2 to 3 years, and then stopped taking this medication of her own accord. She had no hormone replacement therapy for about 2 years, and about 1 year prior to her visit she restarted CEE at a dose of 0.625 mg taken only on alternate days, because she felt that she did not need any more and she experienced symptoms of weight loss, insomnia and other non-specific complaints when she took the medication daily. Her medication at the time of her visit included prednisone, 30 mg/10 mg on alternate days. She had been taking corticosteriods for the past 11 years.

Examination
She weighed 113 lb (51 kg), and had a cushingoid face and an atrophic vagina.

Laboratory Tests
Her estradiol level 24 hours after her last dose of Premarin was 30 pg/mL and her FSH was 74 IU/L. Her bone mineral density scan showed significant risk of fracture both at her spine and at her hip, the t-score in her anterior lumbar spine being −4.0 SD and the t-score for her total hip being −3.83.

Discussion of Case 85

Case 85 has multiple risk factors for bone loss. Removal of one ovary and cyclophosphamide treatment rendered this patient menopausal at the age of 32 years. She was amenorrheic and hypo-estrogenic for 6 years, and only commenced estrogen treatment at the age of 38 years following hysterectomy. Unfortunately, she only took estrogens regularly for 2–3 years. In addition, she had taken constant large doses of glucocorticoids for the treatment of a rheumatologic disorder for 11 years. She was Caucasian and thin, and not surprisingly bone mineral density studies showed significant risk of osteoporotic fracture. This patient had no contraindications to estrogen therapy, but had a multitude of symptoms which she related to estrogens. She should not only be encouraged to take adequate estrogens and calcium, but she was also a candidate for additional agents. For example, she was a candidate for bisphosphonates such as alendronate. Supraphysiologic doses of vitamin D and calcitonin have also been used in the prevention of bone loss following pharmacologic steroid therapy.

THROMBOEMBOLIC DISEASE

Case 86

A 53-year-old patient attended for routine gynecologic examination and to discuss future hormone replacement therapy. Her menarche occurred at age 14 years followed by regular cycles. She had three children, the last at the age of 30 years. She continued with regular cycles, although recently the intervals had become somewhat shorter. Her past history was significant for deep venous thrombosis in the postpartum period of her second pregnancy. She had been treated with heparin and had no problems in her last pregnancy. There was no family history of thromboembolic disease, cancer or osteoporosis, but her father had died of a myocardial infarction at the age of 51 years. She was a non-smoker and only drank alcohol socially. She was not taking any calcium supplements.

Examination
Her weight was 128 lb (58 kg) and her blood pressure was 104/64 mmHg. She was clinically euthyroid, her breasts were fibrocystic and examination was otherwise negative.

Case 87

A 47-year-old patient attended because of hot flashes and night sweats for the previous 18 months. Her menarche occurred at age 11 years, she had regular cycles and she achieved her first pregnancy at the age of 20 years. Following this pregnancy, she had deep vein thrombosis. Over the next 6 years she delivered three other children without complications. She took oral contraceptives for a few years. In the 4 years prior to her visit her menses had become irregular. She smoked 30 cigarettes per day. There was no family history of osteoporosis or ischemic heart disease. Her aunt had had breast cancer in her forties.

Examination
She weighed 108 lb (49 kg) and general examination was normal. Pelvic examination revealed a 4-cm right adnexal mass, which was subsequently found to be a hemorrhagic cyst.

Laboratory Test
Activated partial thromboplastin time was 23.6 seconds (normal range 19–31 seconds), prothrombin time was 11.5 seconds (normal range 10.9–13.4 seconds), lupus anticoagulant was negative, protein C was 157% (normal range 60–150%), protein S was 143% (normal range 56–189%) and antithrombin III was 162 mg/dL (normal range 85–122 mg/dL).

Case 88

A 55-year-old patient attended to discuss hormone replacement therapy. She had had a pregnancy at the age of 21 years and another at the age of 24 years. The second pregnancy was complicated by deep venous thrombosis at 7–8 months' gestation. She took oral contraceptives for 6 years after this pregnancy and had another uneventful pregnancy at the age of 34 years. She had her last menstrual period at the age of 51 years and had not been on hormone replacement therapy. There was no family history of clotting disorders or osteoporosis. She had just been prescribed low-dose thyroid hormone for borderline-low thyroid function.

Examination
She was clinically euthyroid and had a 25-gram goiter. Pelvic examination revealed atrophic vaginal changes.

Laboratory Tests
Bone mineral density studies showed her lumbar spine density to be between –1 and –2.5 SD of mean peak bone mass. Her hip bone mineral density was –2.5 SD of mean peak bone mass – that is, in the osteoporotic range.

Discussion of Cases 86–88

Estrogen therapy (e.g. birth control pill therapy) is contraindicated in women with a past history of thromboembolic disease. Although the dose of estrogens used in postmenopausal women is very small relative to that in birth control pills, prescribing estrogens to women with a past history of venous thrombosis can be problematic. Case 86 represents such a situation. She developed deep venous thrombosis following the high estrogen state of pregnancy, but she also underwent a subsequent pregnancy without ill effects. There was no family history of thromboembolic disease. In addition, she reported a family history of heart disease, and so estrogen therapy could be cardioprotective for her. In such cases it is important to rule out coagulopathies (see discussion of Case 87 below) first, and to discuss the issues involved with the patient. Estrogen therapy is almost always avoided, but in exceptional circumstances, if the decision is made to treat the patient with estrogens, it is important to obtain her informed consent and repeat coagulation parameters on estrogen therapy. Transdermal estrogen, which avoids the first pass through the liver, may be a more suitable form of therapy for such patients, as it may be less likely to affect coagulation parameters. In patients with a history of thromboembolic disease, the use of bisphosphonates should be encouraged to prevent bone loss.

Case 87 presents a similar problem except that she was also a smoker and was encouraged to stop this habit. She had also inadvertently been given oral contraceptives for several years after her deep vein thrombosis. Testing for coagulopathy should include prothrombin time, partial thromboplastin time, lupus anticoagulant, protein C and protein S, and antithrombin III for deficiencies. In addition, one can check for the mutation conferring resistance to activated protein C. These tests are particularly important in patients with family histories of thromboembolic disease or strokes. The finding of such coagulopathies, especially in the face of a family history, would contraindicate estrogen therapy. In Case 88 a deep venous thrombosis had occurred in this patient's second pregnancy. After this event, she had inadvertently been given oral contraceptives for 6 years and even had another (uneventful) pregnancy. Thus although she had had a previous thromboembolic event, she did not experience another such event even under circumstances that placed her at greater risk (namely birth control pills and pregnancy). In addition, she had osteopenia and was likely to become even more osteopenic without estrogen treatment. In her case, the benefits of menopausal estrogen therapy (i.e. its cardiovascular and other benefits, as well as bone maintenance) had to be weighed against the very small increased risk of another thromboembolic event. Bisphosphonates would be suitable for protection against bone loss.

REPLACEMENT THERAPY

Case 89

A 32-year-old patient was seen for hormonal management. Her menarche occurred at the age of 14 years, and she had regular menses. A few months prior to her visit, the finding of a complex, painful, adnexal mass had led to surgery. Severe endometriosis was found, and a hysterectomy and bilateral salpingo-oophorectomy was performed. She had not been placed on estrogen, and was complaining of severe hot flashes and night sweats.

Examination
There were no significant findings.

Discussion of Case 89

Bilateral salpingo-oophorectomy in a young person usually leads to severe hot flashes and night sweats. Unless there is a specific contraindication, such as breast cancer, estrogen therapy is definitely indicated and a dose in the upper menopause replacement-dose range is recommended. For example, 1.25 mg of conjugated equine estrogen or 2 mg of 17 β-estradiol can be given both to alleviate symptoms and to ensure adequate estrogenization in a young person. Patients who have had a hysterectomy do not require progestin therapy, but there are a few exceptions. One of these is following treatment and cure of stage I endometrial cancer, and another is following treatment of severe endometriosis if it involved bladder, bowel or other structures that were not removed at the time of surgery. As endometriotic tissue responds to estrogen, it is possible for unopposed estrogen to lead to hyperplasia and theoretically to cancer.

7

Outflow tract disorders

FIBROIDS

Case 90

A 44-year-old patient was referred because of hot flashes, night sweats and dysmen-orrhea. Her menarche occurred at age 14 years, and she had regular cycles which were initially painful. She had two pregnancies at the ages of 24 and 27 years, and by this time her menstrual pain had improved considerably. At the age of 38 years she had an ectopic pregnancy, at which time a large fibroid was found and removed. During the 2 years prior to her visit her menses had become very painful again, and she had also recently developed hot flashes and night sweats.

Examination
General physical examination was normal. Pelvic examination revealed a 6-week-pregnancy sized uterus. An ultrasound scan was performed.

Laboratory Tests
Her uterus measured 7.3 × 5.3 cm in sagittal view. It contained several fibroids, the largest of which measured 3.6 × 2.8 cm.

Case 91

A 37-year-old patient was referred with a 4-year history of heavy and irregular menstrual cycles with clotting. Her menarche occurred at age 14 years, and she had regular menstrual cycles. She had two uneventful pregnancies at the ages of 28 and 30 years. By the age of 33 years, her menses had become heavy with clots, and she would occasionally experience intermenstrual bleeding. She did not have significant dysmenorrhea. Her mother had had a hysterectomy at the age of 35 years for irregular bleeding.

Examination
She was clinically euthyroid with mild excess hair on her chin. Pelvic examination revealed an enlarged, irregular, retroverted uterus. An endometrial biopsy was performed.

Laboratory Tests
Her hemoglobin was 14 g/dL and her hematocrit was 42%. Her TSH was normal and her prolactin was 5 ng/mL. Ultrasound examination revealed several fibroids, the largest of which measured 4 cm in diameter. Her endometrial biopsy revealed benign secretory endometrium.

POLYPS

Case 92

A 37-year-old patient was referred because of increased menstrual bleeding. She had regular menstrual cycles interrupted by two pregnancies. Over the few years prior to her visit, she had experienced increasingly heavy menses which were painful and contained clots.

Examination
Examination, including a pelvic examination, was unremarkable. A pelvic ultrasound scan was performed.

Laboratory Tests
Ultrasound examination revealed a small hypoechoic lesion within the endometrium, measuring 10 mm in diameter and consistent with an endometrial polyp.

Procedure
A hysteroscopy was performed and the polyp was removed.

Discussion of Cases 90–92

In Case 90, this patient's primary dysmenorrhea had improved following her two pregnancies. Fibroid tumors were diagnosed incidentally and a large one was removed at age 38 years. Although her menses continued to be regular, they had again become very painful in the 2 years prior to her visit and she had menopausal symptoms. Ultrasound examination revealed several fibroid tumors. These are tumors of the muscular wall of the uterus. They are usually multiple and are often the cause of an enlarged, irregular uterus with heavy painful menses. Their growth and maintenance are dependent on estrogen, so they often shrink post-menopausally and they also shrink following GNRH analogue therapy. Although menopause replacement doses of estrogen do not usually lead to major growth of fibroids, they may not shrink either, leading to continuous pain, heavy flow and irregular bleeding patterns. This young perimenopausal patient clearly needed estrogen for relief of her hot flashes and night sweats, but the fibroids were also significantly symptomatic. Thus her best treatment option was a hysterectomy followed by estrogen-only therapy. Despite her relatively young age, given the fact that she was clearly perimenopausal, bilateral oophorectomy was also recommended to avoid the risk of future ovarian cancer.

Uterine fibroids are extremely common, and may be described according to their location (see Figure 7.1). These tumors are virtually always benign, and display slow growth that is estrogen dependent. Signs and symptoms include severe dysmenorrhea, heavy and often prolonged bleeding (possibly with consequent anemia) and not infrequently a uterus that is so enlarged that the fibroids create an abdominal mass. Fibroids may also be associated with miscarriages and less commonly with infertility. Quite often an enlarged fibroid-containing uterus is found in an asymptomatic patient. Fibroids are commonly multiple, and as they are estrogen dependent, they will usually shrink in response to GNRH analogues, but a hypoestrogenic state ensues and thus this is not a permanent solution. Indications for surgery include the above symptoms and anemia. If preservation of reproductive capacity is desired, myomectomy may be performed, although smaller fibroids that are not removed may increase in size, leading to a recurrence of symptoms as in Case 90. Hysterectomy is the definitive treatment, as was subsequently performed in Case 90. Since this patient had already shown signs of perimenopause (hot flashes and night sweats) her ovaries were also removed.

Case 91 also had intermenstrual bleeding, necessitating an endometrial biopsy to rule out endometrial pathology. She was also contemplating surgery and, in view of her age, her ovaries would be left intact. Less commonly, as in Case 92, the patient may present with symptoms that are similar in nature but is subsequently shown to have an endometrial polyp. The polyp presumably interfered with the normal mechanisms of hemostasis.

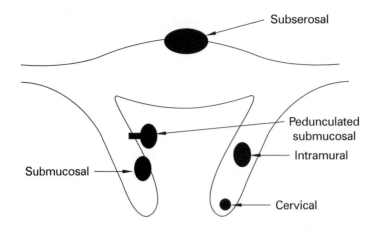

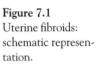

Figure 7.1
Uterine fibroids: schematic representation.

ENDOMETRIOSIS

Case 93

A 37-year-old patient was referred for evaluation of endometriosis. Her menarche occurred at age 16 years, and her cycles were somewhat irregular. Despite this, she achieved pregnancy twice, at the ages of 20 and 26 years. Prior to her second pregnancy, she had become symptomatic with dysmenorrhea and dyspareunia. By the age of 28 years, her symptoms had escalated and a laparoscopy was performed which revealed endometriosis. The lesions were lasered, and she was symptom-free for about 4 years. However, over the subsequent 5 years her symptoms had continued to increase significantly.

Examination
General physical examination was unremarkable. Pelvic examination revealed considerable tenderness, especially over the left adnexa. There was also nodularity in the cul-de-sac. An ultrasound examination was performed.

Laboratory Tests
Ultrasound revealed a normal uterus, a normal left ovary and a 2-cm echogenic cyst in the right ovary.

Case 94

A 29-year-old Asian woman was referred for discussion of the management of endometriosis. Within a few years of her menarche, she had developed severe dysmenorrhea. At the age of 23 years, a laparotomy was performed because of pelvic pain and a pelvic mass. She was found to have stage four endometriosis with an American Society of Reproductive Medicine (ASRM) score of 100. Endometriomas were resected. She received 6-monthly intramuscular injections of Depo-leuprolide, and thereafter she was placed on low-dose oral contraceptives in a continuous fashion. While on this treatment she developed headaches, nausea and paraesthesias. These symptoms resolved when she stopped taking oral contraceptives, but her pelvic pain returned. She had never been pregnant.

Examination
She was extremely thin, weighing 82 lb (37 kg). General physical examination was unremarkable, but pelvic examination revealed a retroverted uterus. In addition, there was a tender area of nodularity in the cul-de-sac. There were no adnexal masses.

Case 95

A 28-year-old patient was referred because of frequent episodes of hemoptysis, which usually occurred on a monthly basis. Her menarche occurred at age 12 years, and she had regular cycles. She achieved pregnancies at the ages of 18, 19 and 23 years. At the age of 24 years, hysterectomy was performed for cancer of the cervix. The ovaries were left intact. Starting at the age of 25 years, she had recurrent episodes of hemoptysis, often with monthly intervals between episodes. Four bronchoscopies and four panendoscopies had failed to reveal the etiology of her bleeding. Some of these episodes were associated with chest pain. She had some pelvic pain prior to her surgery and some dyspareunia, and still occasionally experienced pain on defecation.

Examination
General physical examination was unremarkable. Pelvic examination revealed some adnexal tenderness, but no masses.

Follow-up
She was initially treated with danocrine and subsequently with long-acting gonadotropin-releasing hormone analogs, because of the side-effects she experienced with the danocrine. Her hemoptysis stopped.

Discussion of Cases 93–95

Endometriosis is the finding of endometrial tissue outside the uterus. Numerous theories have been proposed for this condition, the most popular being retrograde menstruation with seeding of endometriosis within the pelvis. Other theories include coelomic transformation and hematogenous spread. Case 93 is a fairly typical case with a history of dysmenorrhea and dyspareunia eventually leading to a laparoscopy. Endometriosis was found and treated by laser vaporization, with subsequent relief of symptoms. As is typical of this disease, the symptoms eventually returned as the endometriosis reappeared. In the absence of a desire for pregnancy, medical treatment can be offered to such patients. These include progestins, oral contraceptives (usually given continuously in order to achieve atrophy), danocrine (a modified androgen which can render the endometriotic tissue atrophic) and finally gonadotropin-releasing hormone agonistic analogs. The analogs cause pituitary desensitization within 7–10 days, thus removing the gonadotropin drive to the ovary. GNRH antagonists are also now available. As endometrial tissue is dependent upon estrogen for its growth, the hypo-estrogenic state that ensues renders the lesions inactive. Unfortunately, loss of estrogens also diminishes bone mass, so prolonged (> 6 months) therapy is not possible unless estrogen and progestins are 'added back' or other agents such as calcitonin or bisphosphonates are used to prevent bone loss. Alternatively, definitive surgery may be offered.

Case 93 opted for the latter and had a hysterectomy and bilateral salpingo-oophorectomy. She subsequently received estrogen therapy. If the endometriosis involves bowel or bladder and is not removed, progestin should also be administered.

Case 94 was a much more severe case with an early age of onset. Her situation was complicated due to the fact that she did not wish to take danocrine and had side-effects while she was on continuous oral contraceptives. A GNRH analog had already been given and was no longer an option because of concern about bone loss, given her extremely thin physique. It is likely that this patient will experience difficulty in conceiving. The infertility of endometriosis relates to scarring of both moderate and severe disease, but even if less severe it may relate to adverse peritoneal factors that may affect fertilization and early embryo development.

Case 95 presented an extremely difficult diagnostic challenge. Recurrent hemoptysis had led to numerous endoscopies. Unfortunately, since this patient had had a hysterectomy, the association of these episodes with menses was not possible. However, the episodes occurred cyclically and endometriosis was eventually suspected. She responded to the hypo-estrogenic state induced by GNRH analogs. Pulmonary endometriosis is one of the possible sites of extrapelvic endometriosis. Other areas include the renal tract and bowel.

MÜLLERIAN AGENESIS

Case 96

An 18-year-old patient was seen because of primary amenorrhea. There was no history of pelvic pain, and secondary sexual characteristics had developed normally. Her past medical history was significant for Kippel–Fiel syndrome. There had been fusion of her neck vertebrae.

Examination
The patient was of normal height and weight. Breast development was normal, and she had normal distribution of pubic and axillary hair. Pelvic examination revealed a blind-ending 2-cm vagina.

Laboratory Tests
Her LH was 7.5 IU/L and FSH was 3.7 IU/L. Pelvic ultrasound examination was performed, and a uterus was not visualized. A 2-cm right ovary was seen as well as a pelvic kidney.

TESTICULAR FEMINIZATION SYNDROME

Case 97

A 20-year-old patient was referred because of primary amenorrhea. Her past history was unremarkable except for a left inguinal hernia repair at the age of 10 years. The details of that surgery were unknown. She experienced a normal growth spurt at the age of 12–13 years and had normal breast development. She had four sisters, three of whom had menstruated. Her fourth sister was amenorrheic at the age of 17 years, like herself. There was no other significant history.

Examination
Her height was 5 feet 3 inches (160 cm). Her breasts were fully developed and there was no galactorrhea. Her pubic and axillary hair were scant, but external genitalia were normal. The vagina ended blindly, and was 7–8 cm in length. No other masses were felt.

Laboratory Tests
Pelvic ultrasound examination did not demonstrate structures which could be compatible with uterus, cervix or ovaries. LH was 16.7 IU/L, FSH was 3.0 IU/L and prolactin was 16.1 ng/mL. DHEA-S was 439 µg/dL, testosterone was 1324 ng/dL (normal male range 300–1200 ng/dL) and estradiol was 23 pg/mL. The karyotype was 46 XY.

Follow-up
Laparoscopy was performed. The right testis measured 2.5 × 2 cm and the left testis measured 3.5 × 1.5 cm, with permanent sutures from previous surgery in the left testis. The uterus, cervix, ovaries and tubes were absent. The testes were removed and estrogen replacement therapy was initiated.

ASHERMAN'S SYNDROME

Case 98

A 36-year-old patient was seen because of secondary amenorrhea of 5 years' duration. After a normal menarche, she had established normal menses and had three term deliveries. She had achieved pregnancy again, had an elective termination at 7 weeks and had remained amenorrheic thereafter. She did not complain of pelvic pain.

Examination
General physical and pelvic examinations were normal, and the patient did not show evidence of thyroid disease.

Laboratory Tests
Thyroid function tests were normal. Her LH was 5.6 IU/L, FSH was 6.2 IU/L and prolactin was 6.1 ng/mL. She was placed on a basal body temperature chart (see Figure 7.2) and the serum progesterone value timed according to the chart was 9.2 ng/mL. A hysterosalpingogram was performed and dye would not pass beyond the cervical canal.

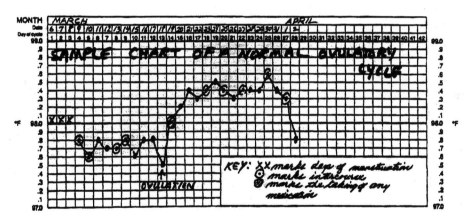

Figure 7.2 Basal body temperature chart: biphasic showing ovulation.

OTHER OUTFLOW TRACT DISORDERS

Case 99

A 21-year-old patient was referred for evaluation of an outflow tract anomaly and also for evaluation of more recent onset menstrual irregularity. Her menarche occurred at age 13 years, and within a few months she settled into monthly cycles that were not painful. She was seen because of some menstrual irregularity, and an outflow anomaly was found. There was no history of diethylstilbestrol exposure, and she had no significant dyspareunia.

Examination

Apart from moderate hirsutism, general examination was unremarkable. Pelvic examination revealed a vaginal septum dividing the vagina into right and left halves. There were two cervices. Ultrasound examination confirmed the presence of two uteri (uterus didelphys).

Case 100

A 35-year-old patient attended to ask for advice about her uterine anomaly. She was totally unaware of a problem until she went into preterm labor at 31 weeks, this being manifested as ruptured membranes. She had a Caesarean section and at this time was noted to have a bicornate uterus, the fetus being in the right horn. A hysterosalpingogram was performed after this pregnancy and showed filling in the right horn only.

Examination
General examination was unremarkable. Pelvic examination revealed an ante-verted uterus which could be felt on the right side only.

Laboratory Tests
The hysterosalpingogram was repeated with slow injection of dye, and again showed filling of dye on the right side only.

Case 101

A 28-year-old patient presented with a 3-year history of infertility. Her past history was unremarkable except for a history of diethylstilbestrol (DES) exposure. Her husband's semen analysis was normal. Her cycles were ovulatory with good mid-luteal progesterone, but her postcoital tests were poor with very scanty mucus production. Other tests had included a hysterosalpingogram which showed a T-shaped uterus (see Figure 7.3), and a laparoscopy which was otherwise normal.

Examination
General examination was unremarkable. Pelvic examination revealed a foreshortened cervix with the characteristic cockscomb deformity seen with DES exposure.

Follow-up
Attempts to correct cervical mucus and achieve pregnancy with estrogen treatment, with and without clomiphene citrate, were unsuccessful. At this time ovulation induction using human menopausal gonadotropins was initiated, the rationale being to improve cervical mucus production by increasing endogenous estrogen levels. Over a 3-year period, the patient received five such courses and pregnancy occurred each time. The first was a biochemical pregnancy, the second was an ectopic pregnancy, the third resulted in a spontaneous vaginal delivery at 38 weeks, and the fourth was heterotopic (i.e. with simultaneous intrauterine and ectopic gestations). The patient miscarried the intrauterine pregnancy before the ectopic one manifested itself. Her last pregnancy was a twin intrauterine pregnancy with spontaneous vaginal delivery at 38 weeks.

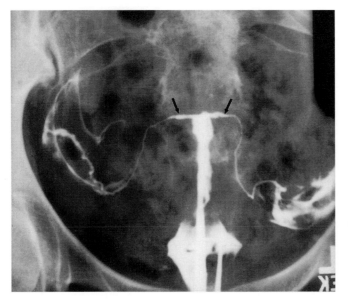

Figure 7.3
Hysterosalpingogram showing a T-shaped uterus (arrows) in a patient with prenatal DES exposure.

Discussion of Cases 96–101

Outflow tract abnormalities may present with reproductive symptoms, or they may be detected incidentally as in Cases 99 and 100. Figure 7.4 shows the more common anomalies that are seen. Case 99 had complete duplication of the internal genitalia, including the vagina, cervix and uterus (uterus didelphys), and this was detected during routine examination. Case 100 had a bicornuate uterus, which was diagnosed during Caesarean section for preterm labor. Patients with this diagnosis face the risk of preterm labor, although after having carried one pregnancy, the chances of the second pregnancy are improved. In this patient's case, only one horn filled with dye at hysterosalpingography; the other horn was assumed to be rudimentary.

Case 101 was a patient with prior diethylstilbestrol (DES) exposure. These patients often have cervical (cockscomb) and uterine (T-shaped) deformities, and may not only experience infertility, as in Case 101, but also be at increased risk for miscarriages, ectopic pregnancies, cervical incompetence and preterm labor. In addition, they are at risk for clear-cell adenocarcinoma of the vagina.

Cases 96 and 97 represent two cases presenting with primary amenorrhea, both with the absence of müllerian structures and a blind-ending vagina, but with very different diagnoses. Both had normal breast development indicative of estrogen exposure. Case 96 had normal distribution of pubic and axillary hair, normal gonadotropins, and an ovary was visualized on ultrasound examination. She represents a case of müllerian agenesis in an otherwise normal female. Renal anomalies are common, as in this case, and the ovaries are functional. Case 97 was also characterized by the absence of müllerian structures, but the lack of pubic hair, very high testosterone levels and the female phenotype are highly suggestive of androgen resistance. Karyotyping showed an XY status, confirming the diagnosis of testicular

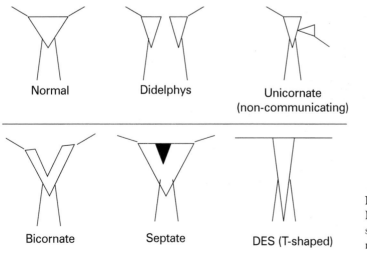

Normal   Didelphys   Unicornate
(non-communicating)

Bicornate   Septate   DES (T-shaped)

Figure 7.4
Müllerian anomalies: schematic representation.

feminization syndrome. The family history is often positive (it may be inherited as an X-linked recessive disorder), as in this case. The lack of müllerian structures is normal under these circumstances because the normal testis will produce müllerian-inhibitory substance in order to get rid of müllerian structures. Figure 7.5 depicts the origin and subsequent development of male and female internal genitalia. These inguinal or abdominal testes are potentially premalignant and need to be removed. Gonadectomy is often delayed in these cases until pubertal development is complete, as apart from lack of menses, these individuals go through an otherwise normal puberty. After surgery, estrogen replacement is essential for bone preservation and cardioprotection.

Case 98 had a normal reproductive history until a pregnancy termination at the age of 31 years. She became amenorrheic at this time and did not experience pelvic pain or other symptoms. Hormonal evaluation was normal. Asherman's syndrome (uterine synechiae or scarring following a curettage, usually in the setting of a pregnancy) was considered, and this was confirmed by the hysterosalpingogram and by her basal body temperature chart, which was biphasic, suggestive of ovulation. Ovulation was subsequently confirmed by a well-timed progesterone value of 9.2 ng/mL. Patients with Asherman's syndrome may present with hypomenorrhea or amenorrhea. Hysterosalpingography often shows the filling defects of scarring (Figure 7.6). Treatment may be effected via hysteroscopy with lysis of scar tissue followed by high-dose estrogen treatment to promote healing. Asherman's syndrome may also lead to recurrent miscarriages.

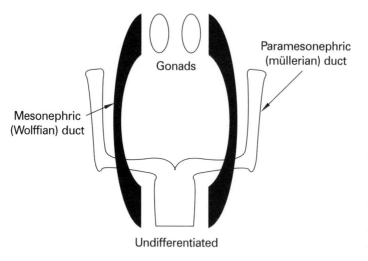

Figure 7.5 Origin and development of male and female reproductive organs: schematic representation. Female: development of müllerian ducts gives rise to uterus, fallopian tubes and part of vagina. Male: development of Wolffian ducts (androgen dependent) gives rise to seminal vesicles, vas deferens and epididymis.

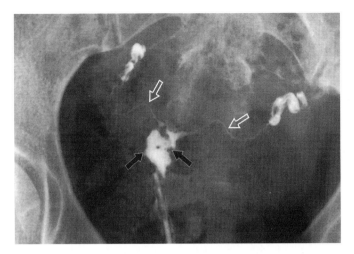

Figure 7.6
Hysterosalpingogram in a patient with Asherman's syndrome showing uterine scarring (closed arrows). The fallopian tubes are normal (open arrows).

8

Infertility

A 28-year-old patient was referred because of secondary infertility. Her menarche occurred at age 12 years, and she had regular cycles with some dysmenorrhea. She took oral contraceptives from the age of 16 to 19 years and achieved pregnancy at the age of 20 years. From the age of 24 to 28 years, she attempted to get pregnant again, without success. Although her partner was different to that of her previous pregnancy, he had fathered a child just before the start of their relationship. Her menses had continued to be regular. Her past medical history included chlamydia infection at the age of 21 years and syphilis at age 25 years. Both conditions had been treated.

Examination
The patient was clinically euthyroid and had a soft 30-gram goiter. Apart from some abdominal hirsutism, examination (including pelvic examination) was normal.

Laboratory Tests
Her mid-luteal progesterone level was 17 ng/mL. A hysterosalpingogram was performed which showed a right hydrosalpinx with some spillage of dye from that side. She also had a small left hydrosalpinx, with no obvious spillage. At laparoscopy both fallopian tubes were found to be bound to the ovaries and their fimbrial ends were not visible. There were filmy adhesions in the cul-de-sac. The adhesions were lysed and fimbrioplasty was performed bilaterally. At the end of the procedure dye was seen to spill freely from both tubes.

Case 103

A 39-year-old patient was referred with a history of secondary infertility involving the same partner. Her menarche occurred at age 12 years and her menstrual cycles were regular. She took oral contraceptives from the age of 17 to 27 years, and became pregnant at the age of 28 years. This pregnancy miscarried. She re-established normal cycles and subsequent attempts at pregnancy were unsuccessful over a 10-year period. She had numerous tests during this time, including two laparoscopies which showed moderate endometriosis. Despite laparoscopic treatment of the endometriosis, numerous clomiphene-stimulated cycles and five cycles of ovulation induction with gonadotropins, she failed to achieve pregnancy.

Examination
General and pelvic examinations did not reveal any abnormalities.

Laboratory Tests
Early cycle FSH was 10 IU/L.

Case 104

A 32-year-old patient attended to seek advice about achieving pregnancy through oocyte donation. Her menarche occurred at age 11 years, and she had essentially regular cycles. At the age of 21 years, inguinal lymphadenopathy led to the diagnosis of Burkitt's lymphoma. Treatment included bilateral oophorectomy followed by 9 months of chemotherapy. She did not receive any irradiation. She was on hormone replacement therapy.

Examination
There were no abnormalities and the uterus was normal.

Case 105

A 37-year-old patient attended for advice regarding her reproductive situation and fertility potential. Her menarche occurred at age 12 years, and she had regular menstrual cycles. At age 36 years, breast cancer was diagnosed and treated surgically. This procedure was both preceded and followed by chemotherapy including cyclophosphamide and adriamycin. The patient also received radiation therapy to her chest post-operatively. Her menses stopped during chemotherapy but had resumed after its completion. She was advised to defer pregnancy for 2 years.

Examination
Examination was normal apart from evidence of breast surgery.

Laboratory Tests
Her day 3 of cycle FSH level was 20.4 IU/L and LH was 6.7 IU/L. Her mid-luteal progesterone level was 7 ng/mL.

Case 106

A 29-year-old man attended with his wife because of infertility of 1 year's duration. His wife gave a history of regular menstrual cycles with some dysmenorrhea which had improved since her menarche. Her mid-luteal progesterone level was high at 19 ng/mL, and she had no abnormal physical findings. Her husband had no past history of orchitis or genitourinary infection.

Examination
The patient was a eugonadal male without gynecomastia or galactorrhea. His testes were of normal size, but he had bilateral varicoceles of moderate size.

Laboratory Tests
His semen analysis was as follows: volume, 3.6 mL; count 16.5 million/mL; motility 45% at 1 hour; excess of severely amorphous sperms. Repeat semen analysis showed a volume of 2.4 mL, count of 31 million/mL and 45% motility. The postcoital test was also abnormal, showing no motile sperm despite adequate cervical mucus.

Follow-up
The patient decided to have varicocelectomy. After 6 months, a repeat semen analysis showed a count of 37 million/mL with a motility of 55%, and his wife became pregnant at this time.

Case 107

A 32-year-old attended because of secondary infertility. Her menarche occurred at age 12 years, and within a few months she had established normal cycles. She achieved her first pregnancy after approximately 2 years of unprotected intercourse. After this pregnancy, she avoided conception for several years, until 1 year prior to her visit. Her cycles continued to be regular. She had some excess hair but no galactorrhea.

Examination
The patient had a 30–35 gram goiter but was not overtly hypothyroid. There was no galactorrhea, and she was mildly hirsute.

Laboratory Tests
Her T_4 was low, her TSH was 56 μIU/mL, and her antithyroglobulin and anti-microsomal antibodies were both positive. A previous serum progesterone measurement on day 25 of her cycle had been 5.4 ng/mL.

Follow-up
She was treated with L-thyroxine and achieved pregnancy within 3 months. She had an uneventful pregnancy.

Case 108

A 31-year-old patient was referred for evaluation of infertility. She had had regular menses since menarche. Her menses were rather painful and this pain had increased slightly over the years. She had attempted pregnancy with a previously fertile partner for 18 months, without success. Her present partner had also been previously fertile, but she had failed to conceive after 1 year of trying. Her past medical history was significant for a ruptured appendix at the age of 2 years.

Examination
Examination, including pelvic examination, did not reveal any abnormalities.

Laboratory Tests
A postcoital test revealed 8 motile sperms/high-power field. Her mid-luteal progesterone level was 13.6 ng/mL. A hysterosalpingogram was obtained and revealed right hydrosalpinx, an open tortuous left tube and a suggestion of loculation of dye on the left side. Laparoscopy revealed extensive pelvic adhesive disease on both sides, and confirmed the right hydrosalpinx.

Discussion of Cases 102–108

Infertility is defined as the inability to achieve pregnancy following 1 year of unprotected intercourse. It is primary (for the individual) if there has been no prior pregnancy (or siring) and secondary if there has. It is best to evaluate the couple together. When obtaining a history and performing a physical examination, attention should be given to delineating potential problems with regard to four major areas or factors that could contribute to infertility. Appropriate tests are described for each factor, and Figures 8.1 and 8.2 outline the evaluation and management of the male and female partners.

1   *Male factor.* An appropriate history of abnormal pubertal development, frequency of shaving, genitourinary infection or surgery, and exposure to chemicals or radiation either occupationally (pesticides) or therapeutically (cancer

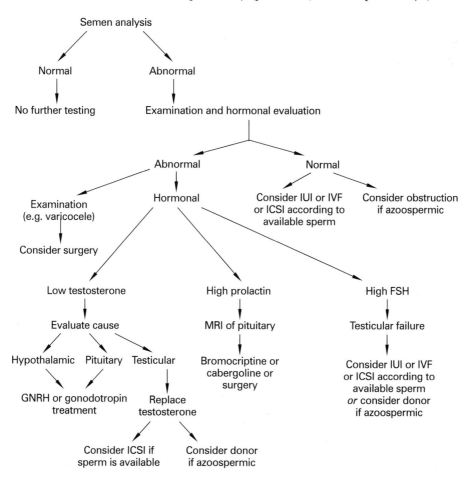

Figure 8.1 Evaluation and management of the infertile couple: *male partner*. IUI, intrauterine insemination; IVF, *in-vitro* fertilization; ICSI, intracytoplasmic sperm injection.

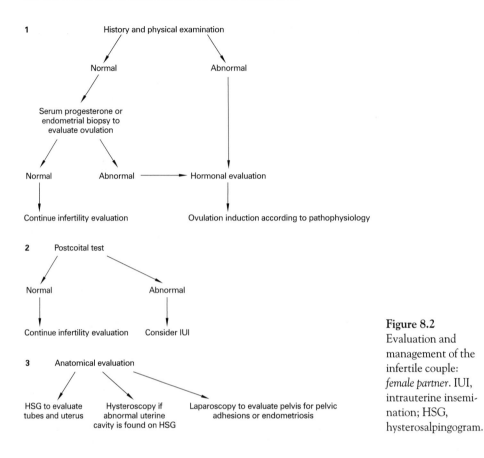

Figure 8.2
Evaluation and management of the infertile couple: *female partner.* IUI, intrauterine insemination; HSG, hysterosalpingogram.

chemotherapy or radiation therapy) should be obtained. Information on coital frequency and ejaculatory difficulty should also be sought. Examination should determine the appropriateness of androgenization (male pattern beard, chest, abdominal and pubic hair), determine testicular size or volume and the presence of varicoceles (virtually always left-sided or bilateral), using a valsalva maneuver, and should also exclude other scrotal abnormalities. A semen analysis must be obtained following 2–4 days of abstinence, and should be examined within 1 hour of collection. A normal semen analysis is as follows:

- volume 1.5–5.0 mL;
- count > 20 million/mL;
- initial motility (< 1 hour) 50%;
- morphology (using Kruger's strict criteria) > 14%;
- in addition, there should be no clumping or significant WBC (< 1 million/mL).

If indicated, serum gonadotropins, testosterone and prolactin levels can be determined. Other tests such as determination of anti-sperm antibodies and the performance of a hamster egg penetration test are also available, but the need for them is best determined by a specialist in infertility.

2   *Cervical factor.* Under normal circumstances, the mucus-producing glands of the cervix respond to estradiol produced by the developing follicles. By mid-cycle (day 13–15), ample clear watery mucus with good stretchability (spinbarkeit) is produced. This is the mucus that is favorable to sperm survival. A small sample of this mucus can easily be removed at mid-cycle following intercourse (2–12 hours later is appropriate), and the number of adequately motile sperm per high-power field is then determined. It should usually exceed 5 sperm/high-power field. Abnormal cervical factor may relate to poor cycle timing, poor mucus production (e.g. due to cervical surgery or inflammation) or an abnormal male factor.

3   *Ovulatory factor.* The topic of ovulatory dysfunction, anovulation or amenorrhea is extensively discussed elsewhere. In women with regular monthly cycles (approximately every 26–30 days), the adequacy of ovulation may be determined by a mid-luteal (day 21–23) progesterone determination. A serum level exceeding 2 ng/mL is indicative of luteinization, but levels of approximately 10 ng/mL or more are desirable. Ovulation may also be determined by an endometrial biopsy, dated by the pathologist, and is usually performed at the end of a cycle. The approximate lengths of the follicular and luteal phases may be determined by a basal body temperature chart (progesterone is thermogenic and elevates the basal temperature, which is obtained upon waking). Figure 7.2 shows a normal ovulatory basal body temperature chart, which is biphasic. In addition, ovulation may also be determined by urinary ovulation monitoring kits which are set to detect the mid-cycle LH surge. Anovulation, ovulatory dysfunction or amenorrhea should be investigated as follows by means of blood tests: LH, FSH, prolactin, thyroid function tests, androgens if appropriate and estradiol if appropriate. Management of ovulatory problems will depend upon the cause. For example, prolactin-producing microadenomas may be treated with bromocriptine, PCOS may be treated using clomiphene citrate (an anti-estrogen that improves the availability of gonadotropins), with or without low-dose glucocorticoids and with or without bromocriptine if there is evidence of adrenal hyperandrogenism or if it is accompanied by hyperprolactinemia, respectively. Patients with major pituitary or hypothalamic disease or PCOS patients who are unresponsive to clomiphene can receive injectable gonadotropins or GNRH (pulsatile treatment).

4   *Anatomical factor.* Infertility may relate to tubal disease, e.g. following pelvic inflammatory disease (PID). It may also relate to intraperitoneal scarring, known as pelvic adhesive disease, from PID or other pathology, such as endometriosis. Endometriosis is the finding of endometrial tissue outside the uterus, and it can present with dysmenorrhea or dyspareunia, but is often asymptomatic. These pockets of tissue may bleed in response to cyclic hormonal stimulation and subsequent withdrawal, and can therefore cause scarring. Even if there is not a significant amount of scarring, endometriosis can lead to infertility through the production of factors or creation of immunologic disturbances that are adverse to ovum pick-up, fertilization and embryogenesis.

In addition, uterine factors such as polyps or endometrial scarring or submu-cosal fibroids (impinging into the uterine cavity) may be associated with infer-tility. Figure 8.3 shows a uterine polyp and Figure 8.4 shows large fibroids distorting the uterine cavity. These and other uterine anomalies are usually also associated with miscarriages. Anatomical factors can be evaluated as follows. First, a hysterosalpingogram will delineate the endometrial cavity and the tubes, outlining their patency and showing the accumulation of fluid in the tubes (hydrosalpinx, as in Figure 8.5 which shows hydrosalpinx on one side and mid-tube obstruction on the other). Secondly, hysteroscopy will demonstrate uterine polyps, submucosal fibroids and scarring, and treatment can be performed at the same time. Thirdly, laparoscopy will show endometriosis, endometriomas (chocolate cysts of the ovaries) and pelvic adhesions. Treatment can usually be given at the time of laparoscopy, but occasionally laparotomy may be necessary.

In infertility evaluation, a fifth factor also occasionally comes into play, namely *aging*, or more specifically the age of the female. Male age is not usually relevant for most couples although it may play a part at extremes of age. Fertility of the female is at its peak in her mid to late twenties, declines after 30 years of age and precipitously so after 35 years, and is greatly impaired after the age of 40 years. An early cycle (day 3) FSH is usually used to delineate ovarian reserve, because the decline in fertility with aging relates to the smaller number and poorer quality of oocytes that remain in the ovary. An FSH of > 12 IU/L is usually a poor prognostic factor.

Case 106 represents a couple with primary infertility. The woman was clearly ovulatory, produced appropriate mucus and gave no history suggestive of anatomical disorders. Her husband had a compromised semen sample (decreased motility and abnormal morphology with or without a compromised count), which was also assumed to be responsible for the abnormal cervical factor. He had bilateral varicoceles.

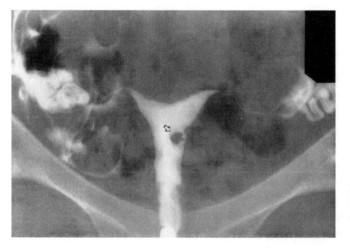

Figure 8.3
Hysterosalpingogram showing a uterine polyp (arrow).

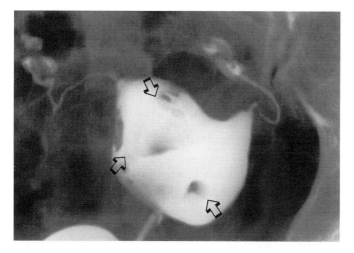

Figure 8.4
Hysterosalpingogram showing distorted uterine cavity (arrows) resulting from fibroids.

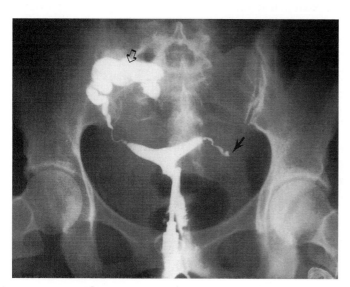

Figure 8.5
Hysterosalpingogram of an infertile patient showing hydrosalpinx (open arrow) and mid-tube obstruction (closed arrows).

Although it would have been reasonable to perform at least a hysterosalpingogram in his wife in order to determine tubal patency, he opted to have a varicocelectomy. This improved his sperm motility and count, and pregnancy resulted a few months post-operatively. Varicoceles are common, and are not always associated with abnormal semen parameters or infertility, and their repair – even when associated with abnormal parameters – does not always lead to an improvement in semen parameters or pregnancy. None the less, many patients have had favorable results. The mechanism of varicocele-induced compromised semen quality is poorly understood and may relate to higher intratesticular temperatures.

Cases 102 and 108 represent tubal disease related to previous pelvic inflammatory diseases. Although Case 102 had such a past history, Case 108 did not. However, the patient in Case 108 gave a history of ruptured appendix at the age of

2 years, which may have led to the subsequent tubal and pelvic disease. Case 102 was treated at the time of laparoscopy. After allowing a reasonable time for pregnancy to occur, while ensuring normal ovulations and normal sperm survival, assisted reproduction (*in-vitro* fertilization and embryo transfer) would be the next appropriate treatment to be offered. In the event of natural pregnancy, careful testing with HCG determinations and ultrasound examination would be necessary to exclude an ectopic pregnancy. Case 108 was not amenable to laparoscopic treatment. Case 108 was suitable for *in-vitro* fertilization and embryo transfer following her initial surgical evaluation.

Case 105 had two reasons for poor ovarian reserve, namely her age and, in particular, her previous chemotherapy. This was reflected by her elevated FSH level. Her prognosis for fertility was poor. Donor oocytes (if pregnancy after her breast cancer treatment was indeed deemed to be reasonable) or adoption were the two reasonable alternatives for this patient. Case 104, with bilateral oophorectomy at age 21 years, was clearly a suitable candidate for oocyte donation. During this procedure, donor oocytes are fertilized with the recipient's husband's sperm, and the resulting embryos are transferred into a hormonally prepared recipient uterus.

Case 103 had achieved a spontaneous pregnancy at 28 years of age, but had thereafter failed to become pregnant. Endometriosis seemed to be her major infertility factor. Despite surgical treatment, followed by intensive ovulation induction using clomiphene and later gonadotropins, she had failed to become pregnant. Her next reasonable option was *in-vitro* fertilization and embryo transfer. During this procedure, the development of multiple oocytes is stimulated using injectable gonadotropins. Figure 8.6 represents an ultrasound examination depicting multifollicular recruitment. These follicles are retrieved via ultrasound-guided follicular aspiration and fertilized *in vitro* using the husband's sperm. The resulting embryos (usually less than 4) are transferred into the uterus. Any surplus embryos can be cryopreserved for future use. This patient's age and FSH of 10 IU/L are cause for concern and are likely to diminish her chances of conception and a successful pregnancy.

Case 107 had primary hypothyroidism and a relatively low mid-luteal progesterone level, and achieved pregnancy within 3 months of thyroid hormone replacement. Thyroid disease has been associated with decreased fertility and increased miscarriage rate. It is readily treatable, and so should be treated prior to initiation of a pregnancy. Both primary hypothyroidism and hyperthyroidism have been associated with ovulatory dysfunction. Primary hypothyroidism may lead to hyperprolactinemia and galactorrhea through excess thyrotropin-releasing hormone (TRH)-mediated prolactin stimulation. TRH stimulates both TSH and prolactin production and release. Excess prolactin can lead to ovulatory disturbances.

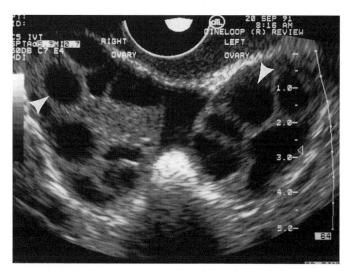

Figure 8.6
Endovaginal ultrasound examination of ovaries in an infertile patient undergoing controlled ovarian hyperstimulation. Multifollicular recruitment is shown (arrows).

9

Recurrent spontaneous abortion

A 33-year-old patient was referred because of three consecutive pregnancy losses over the preceding 2 years. Her menarche occurred at age 14 years, and she had regular menstrual cycles. At the age of 24 years she had her first pregnancy, with an uncomplicated delivery at term. She had continued with regular menses and over the previous 2 years had established three pregnancies, with a different partner, but all three had resulted in miscarriages at 6 or 9 weeks' gestation. She had dilatation and curettage performed after her second miscarriage. At the age of 29 years she was diagnosed with Hashimoto's thyroiditis and hypothyroidism. Her antimicrosomal antibodies were strongly positive and she had been taking thyroxine since that time.

Examination
The patient was clinically euthyroid, with a palpable thyroid. Examination was otherwise unremarkable.

Laboratory Tests
Thyroid function tests were normal, and her mid-luteal progesterone level was 14.9 ng/mL. Her glucose and glycohemoglobin levels were in the normal non-diabetic range. Her partial thromboplastin time was normal at 28.8 seconds, her platelet count was normal, and her lupus anticoagulant was negative, as were her anticardiolipin (IgG and IgM) antibodies. Karyotyping of the patient and her husband was requested but was not performed.

Follow-up
She achieved pregnancy again but had some spotting at 5 weeks. Her serum progesterone level was 16 ng/mL and an intrauterine gestational sac was seen. She was treated with natural progesterone. The remainder of her pregnancy was uneventful and she delivered at term.

Case 110

A 26-year-old patient was referred because of recurrent miscarriages. Her menarche occurred at age 17 years, and her cycles had been irregular, up to 45 days apart. Her first pregnancy was at the age of 22 years, and she had four consecutive pregnancy losses, all involving the same partner.

Examination
The patient was clinically euthyroid and did not have hirsutism or galactorrhea. Pelvic examination was normal.

Laboratory Tests
The following tests were all normal: glucose and thyroid function tests, antiphospholipid antibodies, antithyroid antibodies, lupus anticoagulant, hysteroscopy and karyotyping of both partners. Cervical *myocoplasma hominis* cultures were positive and the patient was treated with antibiotics. Her testosterone level was 41 ng/dL, DHEA-S was 309 μg/dL and prolactin was 5 ng/mL. A day 20 of cycle progesterone measurement was < 1 ng/mL.

Case 111

A 41-year-old patient attended because of recurrent miscarriages. Her menarche occurred at age 15 years, and she had regular cycles. From the ages of 18–38 years she took oral contraceptives and resumed 28-day cycles. Her first pregnancy was at the age of 39 years, but she miscarried at 8 weeks. Six months later, she miscarried at 6 weeks. Again, 6 months later pregnancy was diagnosed by beta-human chorionic gonadotropin (HCG) determination at the time of her expected menses. A serum progesterone measurement at this time was low at 2.3 ng/mL, and she miscarried the next day. She had one other biochemical pregnancy prior to her visit, and by this time her cycles were becoming shorter (approximately 25 days apart).

Examination
The patient was clinically euthyroid and had no goiter. Breast and pelvic examinations were unremarkable.

Laboratory Tests
Her early-cycle FSH level was 10 IU/L. A day 21 of cycle progesterone measurement was 11.5 ng/mL, but her cycle was only 24 days in duration. Thyroid function tests, antithyroid antibodies, lupus anticoagulant, anticardiolipin antibodies and serum glucose were all normal. A hysterosalpingogram was normal, as was her karyotype (her husband had previously fathered a child and did not have a karyotype).

Follow-up
She was given clomiphene, 50 mg for 5 days, and had a progesterone level of 26.6 ng/mL in a 27-day cycle. Unfortunately, she became pregnant again in a non-clomiphene cycle, and had a beta-HCG level of 407 mIU/mL together with a progesterone level of 1.3 ng/mL on day 31 of her cycle. This pregnancy was supplemented with oral natural progesterone, given in the form of lozenges, and she carried her pregnancy to term.

Case 112

A 35-year-old patient was referred with a history of four recurrent miscarriages. Her menarche and subsequent menses were normal. She had had an uneventful pregnancy 11 years prior to her visit, and since that time she had miscarried four pregnancies. A comprehensive work-up, including karyotyping of both partners and a hysterosalpingogram, had revealed normal results. However, antiphospholipid antibodies had been positive.

Examination

The patient was clinically euthyroid and had no goiter. Apart from mild hirsutism, a general physical examination was unremarkable.

Case 113

A 35-year-old patient was referred because of three consecutive miscarriages. Her menarche occurred at age 11 years, she established normal cycles, and from the age of 24–29 years she took oral contraceptives. Shortly thereafter, she became pregnant and had an uneventful pregnancy. She returned to taking oral contraceptives until the age of 31 years. She then had three consecutive miscarriages over the course of the next 3 years, and required dilatation and curettage for two of these. Her cycles continued to be regular and with normal flow.

Examination
The patient was clinically euthyroid and did not have a goiter. General physical and pelvic examinations were unremarkable.

Laboratory Tests
Her thyroid function tests were normal and her mid-luteal progesterone level was 22.3 ng/mL. Her fasting glucose and glycosylated hemoglobin levels were normal. Her early-cycle FSH was 4.3 IU/L. Her prothrombin time and partial thromboplastin time were normal. Her antinuclear antibody (ANA) was negative, as were tests for lupus anticoagulants and anticardiolipin antibodies. A hysterosalpingogram showed a normal uterine cavity with bilateral spillage of dye. Karyotyping of both partners was recommended but was not performed.

Case 114

A young couple attended to discuss recent tests pertaining to a history of recurrent miscarriages. Two consecutive pregnancies had resulted in a miscarriage. The second conceptus was examined and found to have a chromosomal abnormality (an extra chromosome 8 was found), leading to karyotype examination of the parents.

Laboratory Tests

The husband's karyotype revealed a normal male pattern of 46 XY. His wife had a balanced translocation 46XX, t(2;8) (q21; q31).

Case 115

A 33-year-old patient was referred because of a history of recurrent miscarriages involving the same partner. Her menarche occurred at age 11 years, and her menses were always irregular. She had a miscarriage at the age of 28 years, followed by a full-term pregnancy at age 29 years. She had two other miscarriages at the age of 32 and 33 years, respectively. In between pregnancies she was oligomenorrheic. Her first and second miscarriages had required dilatation and curettage, but there had been no change in menstrual flow. She also had a history of hirsutism.

Examination
The patient was clinically euthyroid and had no goiter. She was mildly hirsute. Pelvic examination revealed a retroverted uterus.

Laboratory Tests
Her LH was 67 IU/L, FSH was 6.7 IU/L (when oligomenorrheic), prolactin was 12.2 ng/mL and thyroid function tests were normal. Her ANA, lupus anticoagulant and antithyroid antibodies were negative. Her testosterone and DHEA-S levels 6 weeks after her miscarriage were 33.5 ng/dL and 95.7 µg/dL, respectively.

Follow-up
She was treated with an oral contraceptive for 1 month, followed by clomiphene citrate, and achieved pregnancy during the second cycle of treatment. She then had a full-term pregnancy.

Discussion of Cases 109–115

Spontaneous abortion is the most common complication of pregnancy, occurring in 10–15% of pregnant women. In approximately 3–5% of women it occurs repeatedly. Traditionally, evaluation and therapy have been offered to women with three or more spontaneous abortions, so called 'habitual-aborters'. Evaluation of a *pregnant* woman with previous multiple miscarriages should include early ultrasonographic evaluation for fetal cardiac activity and fetal heart rate, presence or otherwise of the embryo, and gestational sac appearance. If the woman miscarries, it is important to obtain a karyotype of the conceptus material. In a habitual aborter without a current pregnancy, investigations should be performed and these are outlined in Box 9.1. General and special chemistry tests should rule out diabetes, thyroid disease and major renal and liver diseases. Endocrine studies should determine the normalcy of the menstrual cycle, with special emphasis on the length and strength of the luteal phase (as determined by basal body temperature charts, serum progesterone levels and endometrial biopsy). If the luteal phase is abnormal, other tests, including prolactin, androgens and gonadotropins, should be performed. Early-cycle (day 3) FSH may help to delineate ovarian reserve (ovarian aging). An abnormally high LH/FSH ratio suggests polycystic ovary syndrome (hypersecretion of LH has been associated with spontaneous abortion), and serum androgens may be concomitantly elevated. Autoimmune disease is a risk factor for pregnancy loss, and ANA, lupus anticoagulant and anticardiolipin antibodies should be determined, as well as a partial thromboplastin time. Antithyroid antibodies have also recently been implicated. Infectious agents have been implicated in pregnancy loss, including *Chlamydia*, *Ureaplasma urealyticum* and bacterial vaginosis. Although there are no conclusive data linking these infections with miscarriages, there is some support for antimicrobial therapy. Uterine anomalies and cervical incompetence are observed in more than 15% of patients who experience recurrent pregnancy loss. Uterine anomalies include intrauterine adhesions, fibroids, uterine septum and bicornate uterus. Other putative factors include the presence of endometriosis, a defective hemostatic response to pregnancy and allo-immunologic mechanisms (elevated levels of natural killer cells have been found in the blood and uterus of women with spontaneous abortions of karyotypically normal pregnancies). Finally, parental karyotyping may reveal chromosomal anomalies, such as balanced translocations, that may lead to aneuploidy and recurrent pregnancy loss.

Box 9.1 Evaluation of recurrent pregnancy loss

Renal function
Liver function
Glucose and hemoglobin A_1C
Thyroid function tests, including TSH and antithyroid antibodies
Progesterone: mid-luteal*
Endometrial biopsy for dating*
Chlamydia and *Ureaplasma urealyticum* cultures
ANA, lupus anticoagulant and anticardiolipin antibodies
Hysterosalpingogram or hysteroscopy to delineate uterine anomalies, adhesions, fibroids or polyps
Parental karyotyping

*If abnormal (progesterone < 6 ng/mL or biopsy out of phase by > 2 days), a full hormonal evaluation should be performed to determine the cause.

In Case 109, a previous full-term pregnancy ruled out major congenital uterine anomalies and made a chromosomal abnormality in the mother less likely, Paternal chromosomes were not obtained. An immune mechanism was possible, given the patient's strongly positive antimicrosomal antibodies. Although she had no evidence of luteal insufficiency when evaluated pre-pregnancy, she was treated with progesterone in early pregnancy because her serum progesterone level at that time was somewhat lower than is usually seen in pregnancy (> 20 ng/mL). Case 110 clearly had ovulatory dysfunction based on hyperandrogenism, and that may have been the cause of her recurrent miscarriages. She also had evidence of mycoplasma infection. Case 111 was an older patient with recurrent miscarriages. Previous laboratory evaluation in very early pregnancy had revealed a healthy serum HCG but a low progesterone level (2.3 ng/mL). When she accidentally became pregnant again, in a non-treatment cycle, she again displayed luteal insufficiency with a progesterone level of 1.3 ng/mL. Remarkably, with progesterone supplementation that pregnancy went to term.

Case 112 had had a previous normal pregnancy and there was no discernible cause of the recent recurrent miscarriages apart from positive antiphospholipid antibodies. In the antiphospholipid syndrome, the most specific type of pregnancy loss is usually fetal death, often in the second and early third trimester.

Case 113 had previously had a full-term pregnancy with her partner, but had subsequently had three consecutive miscarriages. No obvious cause was found for the miscarriages. Karyotyping was recommended because it was possible, despite the previous normal pregnancy, for one partner to have a balanced translocation.

In Case 114, chromosomal examination of the conceptus led to parental karyotyping which revealed a balanced translocation in the female partner.

Case 115 had a history of oligomenorrhea dating from menarche, and although elevated androgens were not demonstrated (possibly because she was just recovering from a miscarriage), her very high LH:FSH ratio was pathognomonic for polycystic ovary syndrome. There is now substantial evidence linking high LH levels (certainly an LH value of 67 IU/L is extremely high) and miscarriages. This patient was deliberately given an oral contraceptive (to lower the LH levels), and ovulation was then immediately induced with clomiphene citrate, leading to consecutive ovulatory cycles. She achieved pregnancy in the second cycle, and this pregnancy went to term.

Male disorders

Case 116

A 51-year-old man was referred for evaluation of left breast enlargement of 1 year's duration. A few months previously he had been evaluated for abdominal pain, and computerized scanning had shown a tumor in the tail of his pancreas. This was resected, but he had evidence of metastatic disease. His past history was significant for right orchiectomy at the age of 21 years.

Examination
The patient was euthyroid. Mildly tender subareolar tissue was found in his left breast. His left testis was normal.

Laboratory Tests
His testosterone level was 797 ng/dL (normal range 300–1200 ng/dL), prolactin was 7 ng/mL, estradiol was 52 pg/mL and HCG was 17.7 IU/L. Immunostaining of the pancreatic tumor was positive for HCG.

Discussion of Case 116

Gynecomastia is a common clinical condition, especially in pubertal boys when transient proliferation of the ducts and surrounding mesenchymal tissue takes place. This usually involutes, but it may remain if there is a relative imbalance between estrogen and androgen levels. Alterations in the ratio of estrogen to androgen can be found in a number of circumstances, as outlined below.

1   Physiologic circumstances:
   - neonatal;
   - pubertal;
   - involutional (older males).
2   Pathologic circumstances:
   - neoplasms:
     (i)   testicular (germ cell, Leydig or Sertoli)
     (ii)   adrenal
     (iii) ectopic production of human chorionic gonadotropin (e.g. lung cancer);
   - primary gonadal failure (Klinefelter's);
   - secondary hypogonadism;
   - androgen-insensitivity syndromes (incomplete);
   - liver and renal disease;
   - hyperthyroidism;
   - medications (chemotherapy (alkylating agents), anabolic steroids, HCG, anti-androgens, isoniazid, ketoconazole, digoxin, H_2 blockers, phenothiazines, marijuana).

Case 116 had a past history of a testicular tumor leading to orchiectomy. Years later a metastatic pancreatic tumor secreting HCG was found. He had a normal testosterone level and a mildly elevated estradiol level. Unilateral gynecomastia may represent a stage in the development of bilateral disease. Evaluation by history and careful physical examination may reveal the cause. Laboratory tests should include measurements of LH, FSH, testosterone, estradiol, HCG, thyroid function tests and prolactin. Treatment, if necessary, varies according to the cause. Offending drugs should be discontinued if possible. Surgical therapy is definitive, but the gynecomastia may also respond to anti-estrogen, such as clomiphene citrate or tamoxifen and to aromatase inhibitors (inhibiting aromatization of androgens to estrogens), such as testolactone.

Case 117

A 27-year-old man was evaluated for primary infertility. His wife had been seen initially, and during the course of infertility work-up his semen analysis had shown that he was azoospermic. His pubertal development had been normal until the age of 14 years. At this time, he remembers having a painful left testicular swelling. His past medical history was otherwise not significant. He recalled never having had much body hair, and he shaved every 2 weeks. His recent job had involved exposure to benzene and styrene.

Examination
The patient was clinically euthyroid and had slight gynecomastia but no galactorrhea. He had diminished facial hair, absence of chest hair and a female escutcheon. Both testes were small, firm and measured 1.5 × 1 × 0.75 cm. He had no varicocele.

Laboratory Tests
LH was 20 IU/L, FSH was 29.5 IU/L, prolactin was 8.3 ng/mL, testosterone was 250 ng/dL (normal male range > 300 ng/dL) and TSH was 1.1 μIU/mL.

Case 118

A 31-year-old man attended with his wife to discuss fertility issues. He had been diagnosed with Hodgkin's disease at the age of 15 years and had received cyclophosphamide and vincristine over a period of 2 years. Fourteen years later, recurrent nodal disease necessitated further chemotherapy, and he was treated with six cycles of adriamycin and lomustine. Prior to this latest round of chemotherapy, he had collected four ejaculates for cryopreservation. These revealed counts of 3.2, 4.7, 21.5 and 5 million/mL, respectively. The motilities were in the range 43–63%. The patient became azoospermic after the most recent round of treatment.

Case 119

A 45-year-old man was referred because of oligospermia. He had originally presented to a physician because his wife had failed to conceive after 2 years of exposure to pregnancy. Multiple semen analysis had revealed counts of approximately 15 million/mL with motilities of 30–40%. He had received clomiphene citrate treatment but there was no improvement in his semen parameters. He had been found to have a significant left varicocele and, in view of the above situation, he had a varicocelectomy performed 15 months prior to his visit.

Examination
The patient was clinically euthyroid and well masculinized. His testes were within normal size limits, the right one being slightly larger than the left.

Laboratory Tests
His FSH was 9.4 IU/L (normal range 1–8 IU/L), testosterone was 347 ng/dL and prolactin was 12 ng/mL. His semen analysis 15 months post-varicocelectomy was as follows: volume, 1.0 mL; count, 11.75 million/mL; 27% motility within the first hour; 94% normal morphology (old morphologic criteria, normal > 50%).

Case 120

A 33-year-old man was referred because of secondary infertility. Renal disease had been diagnosed at the age of 17 years. He had a renal transplant at the age of 30 years and again at age 32 years because of rejection. His second kidney was working well and he had a normal serum creatinine level. Seven years prior to his visit, his wife had established a pregnancy which unfortunately miscarried. His medication consisted of cyclosporine and prednisone.

Examination
The patient was clinically well androgenized, had no gynecomastia or galactorrhea, and general examination was unremarkable. He had a large right hydrocele, and his left testis was within normal size limits.

Laboratory Tests
Two semen samples revealed azoospermia. His LH was 4.3 IU/L, FSH was 1.4 IU/L, prolactin was 6.6 ng/mL, testosterone was 343 ng/dL, estradiol was 64 pg/mL (normal range < 50 pg/mL) and TSH was normal.

Follow-up
Testicular biopsy confirmed obstructive azoospermia.

Discussion of Cases 117–120

Normal reproductive function in the male depends on the integrity of the hypo-thalamic–pituitary–testicular axis. As in the female, the hypothalamus produces GNRH in a pulsatile fashion, leading to synthesis and release of the gonadotropins LH and FSH. LH affects testosterone synthesis by testicular Leydig cells. In the presence of sufficient intratesticular testosterone concentrations, the seminiferous tubules respond to FSH, and germ-cell growth and development leads to the production of mature spermatozoa. These spermatozoa are stored within the epididymis and are released during ejaculation through the vas deferens and subse-quently the urethra. Figure 10.1 outlines the hypothalamic–pituitary–testicular axis.

Case 117 represents primary testicular failure (as evidenced by high FSH and LH levels). Although this may have been related to severe orchitis sustained in early puberty, the patient's small testes also raise the possibility of Klinefelter's syndrome, which would present in exactly this manner. Not only were the seminiferous tubules affected, but there was also impairment of Leydig-cell function as evidenced by scant body hair, slight gynecomastia and low serum testosterone levels. In Klinefelter's syndrome, the karyotype would be XXY. Although recent occupa-tional exposure to toxic chemicals was also reported, his history pre-dated such exposure, which in any case was unlikely to lead to small testes.

Case 118 had received multiple chemotherapy, including agents known to induce testicular failure, such as cyclophosphamide. Sterility is a well-known complication of cancer therapy in both males and females. Although this patient was not azoospermic prior to his second round of chemotherapy, his sperm counts

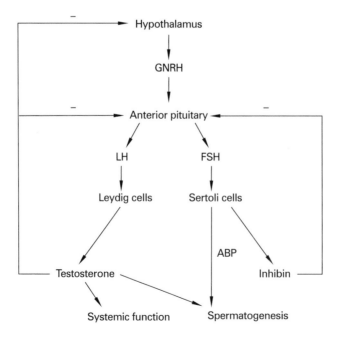

Figure 10.1
Hypothalamic–pituitary–testicular axis. ABP, androgen-binding protein.

were very significantly impaired and were unlikely to yield sufficient numbers of motile sperm for routine insemination post-thaw. Provision would have to be made for assisted reproduction in such a case. If the numbers were sufficient post-thaw, fertilization of his wife's oocytes *in vitro* could be attempted. Alternatively, intracytoplasmic sperm injection could be attempted using single spermatozoa.

Case 119 had oligoasthenospermia (low count and motility) and had been unable to impregnate his wife. He also had a left varicocele. Varicoceles are not infrequently associated with abnormal semen parameters and, under such circumstances, surgical correction is usually suggested. Quite frequently the abnormal parameters improve and pregnancy occurs, but not in every case. In Case 119, despite varicocelectomy, this patient's semen parameters remained abnormal. Although the precise mechanism is not known, it may be related to a high intratesticular temperature, which may be inhibitory to spermatogenesis. Occasionally, patients with oligoasthenospermia are also treated with clomiphene citrate, as this patient was. The object of clomiphene is to improve the availability of gonadotropins. However, since lack of gonadotropins is not usually the cause of defective spermatogenesis, it does not often result in an improvement of semen parameters.

Case 120 also presented with infertility. His wife had previously achieved pregnancy, but unfortunately she had miscarried. The patient had undergone two renal transplants, the second one being successful. Although impaired renal function may decrease gonadal function reversibly, leading to both altered sperm production and a hypogonadal state (diminished testosterone levels), his renal function was normal at the time of his visit. The mechanism of reproductive disturbance in patients with renal disease is complex, affecting both hypothalamic and gonadal function. This patient was well androgenized and had a normal left testis (the right testis could not be felt because of a hydrocele). He was azoospermic but had normal gonadotropins, prolactin and testosterone levels. Review of his surgical records revealed extensive scarring and obstructive azoospermia.

Special cases

Case 121

A 35-year-old man complained of diminished sex drive and decreased potency of recent onset. Additional history included a diminished frequency of shaving, and headaches. He had previously fathered a child, now aged 4 years.

Examination
His weight was 256 lb (116 kg) and his blood pressure was 122/70 mmHg. He was clinically euthyroid and had no goiter. Body hair distribution was of male pattern, and the amount was within normal limits. He had no galactorrhea or gynecomastia, and examination of his visual fields and fundi did not reveal any abnormalities. His testes measured approximately $4.5 \times 3 \times 1.5$ cm (normal size), but were somewhat soft in consistency.

Laboratory Tests
Testosterone was 139 ng/dL, LH was 3.5 IU/L, FSH was 2.8 IU/L, prolactin was 447 ng/mL, T_4 was 7.1 μg/dL, TSH was 1.0 μIU/mL, cortisol was 14.2 μg/dL (a.m.), growth hormone was 1.1 ng/mL and somatomedin C (I_gF-I) was 148 ng/mL (normal range, 123–463 ng/mL) MRI showed an 8-mm non-enhancing mass in the pituitary gland on the right side.

Discussion of Case 121

This patient's diagnosis was clearly a prolactin-producing pituitary adenoma. As in women, prolactin in excess shuts off the hypothalamic–pituitary–testicular axis (its main effect is on hypothalamic GNRH production), resulting in hypogonadism. This man's low serum testosterone level was due to diminished availability of LH, and resulted in decreased libido and potency. Hyperprolactinemia itself has been associated with erectile dysfunction. He responded to dopamine agonist suppression of prolactin.

There are three major pathways of erection, namely reflexogenic (tactile stimulation), psychogenic and nocturnal during REM sleep. Erection involves the co-ordinated interactions of nerves, muscles and blood vessels. In the flaccid state, the corporeal smooth muscle is contracted, with little blood flow into the penis. Nerve impulses release neurotransmitters, causing vasodilatation, and the corporeal sinuses fill with blood. The causes of erectile dysfunction include the following.

1   *Psychogenic causes*: affect 10–30% of impotent men.
2   *Endocrinologic causes*: as in the above case, androgen deficiency impairs sexual interest and may reduce potency. Prolactin excess may also be associated with erectile dysfunction, and sexual function may not improve with testosterone replacement alone in such patients. The role of androgens in erection is not entirely clear.
3   *Neurogenic causes*: spinal cord disorders and peripheral neuropathies secondary to alcoholism, vitamin B deficiency, and diabetes may lead to neurogenic erectile dysfunction.
4   *Arteriogenic causes*: a common mechanism and usually related to arteriosclerosis itself, often associated with diabetes, hypertension, hyperlipidemia and smoking.
5   *Drug-induced causes*: antihypertensives including thiazide diuretics, beta-blockers, methyldopa, clonidine, reserpine and guanethidine. Antidepressants and antipsychotic agents may also lead to erectile dysfunction.
6   *Cavernosal factors*: failure of the venous closure mechanism, necessary for the trapping of blood within the erect penis, may also lead to erectile dysfunction.

Case 122

A 43-year-old patient was referred because of irregular menses. Her menarche occurred at age 13 years, and she had regular menstrual cycles interrupted by two pregnancies at the ages of 28 and 32. She continued with regular menses until 4 months prior to her visit. During this time they were irregular, often with two periods in 1 month. Her past medical history was significant for an abdominal desmoid tumor, which was diagnosed and resected at age 37 years. Unfortunately, the tumor recurred, leading to a second bowel resection. In the 18 months prior to her visit, she had received tamoxifen, 10 mg twice daily, as desmoids have been known to respond to this therapy.

Examination
The patient was clinically euthyroid and general physical examination was unremarkable. Pelvic examination revealed a slightly enlarged uterus. Pelvic ultrasound examination and endometrial biopsy were performed.

Laboratory Tests
Pelvic ultrasound examination revealed a slightly enlarged uterus containing several small fibroids, the largest of which was 2.5 cm in diameter. A 5-cm right ovarian cyst was also identified. The endometrial stripe was 11 mm in diameter. Endometrial biopsy showed early adenomatous hyperplasia. TSH, prolactin and and hemoglobin levels were all normal. Serum estradiol, on day 11 of the patient's cycle, was 877 pg/mL.

Discussion of Case 122

Tamoxifen is an anti-estrogen but it also has estrogenic properties, and these two properties vary from one tissue to another. Its anti-estrogenic properties form the basis of its use in the treatment of estrogen-receptor-positive postmenopausal breast cancer. During such use it may stimulate endometrial growth through its estrogenic properties. This is illustrated by the patient in Case 122, who developed early adenomatous hyperplasia in response to tamoxifen. She was premenopausal and her very high follicular-phase estradiol was also presumably related to tamoxifen stimulation of gonadotropin production and subsequent ovarian stimulation. Sustained high estrogen concentrations serve to further stimulate the endometrium in such patients. Ovarian cyst development has also been described in patients on anti-estrogens.

Case 123

A 26-year-old patient was referred with a 14-month history of secondary amenorrhea. Menarche occurred at the age of 17 years, and thereafter her periods were irregular, occurring every 6 weeks to 3 months. At the age of 18 years she had a laparoscopy and large ovaries were found. Her periods continued to occur at irregular intervals, and from time to time she was given medroxyprogesterone acetate to induce one. At the age of 22 years, she had an unexpected pregnancy. This pregnancy manifested itself by 4 weeks of continuing bleeding. Dilatation and curettage (D&C) was performed, but she continued to bleed, so another D&C was performed. At this point, the diagnosis of an ectopic pregnancy was made. She had a laparotomy and the tube was saved. After the pregnancy, the patient received oral contraceptives for a few months, these being followed by light periods. After discontinuing the contraceptives, she became essentially amenorrheic with only three or four light periods over an interval of 2 years. Another laparoscopy was performed and large polycystic ovaries were found. Over the subsequent year or so she received four courses of medroxyprogesterone acetate, but she failed to have any periods. She therefore attended the endocrine clinic because of the above history of menstrual irregularity dating from the menarche and culminating in 14 months of amenorrhea. She also complained of hirsutism and weight gain.

Examination
She was moderately overweight at 178 lb (81 kg) and was also moderately hirsute but not virilized. She had no galactorrhea, and pelvic examination revealed a partly open cervical os with extrusion of moderate amounts of clear, thin mucus.

Laboratory Tests
Prolactin was 13 ng/mL, testosterone was 69 ng/dL, DHEA-S was 420 μg/dL, estradiol was 103 pg/mL, LH was 6 IU/L and FH was 12 IU/L (normal up to 20 IU/L).

Discussion of Case 123

This patient had PCOS as evidenced by the following features:

1 irregular menses dating from the menarche;
2 an initial endometrial response to medroxyprogesterone acetate (MPA) challenge (shedding of the endometrium following treatment);
3 elevated testosterone and DHEA-S with mid-follicular levels of estradiol;
4 evidence of adequate estrogenization clinically as judged by cervical mucus examination;
5 evidence of polycystic ovaries at laparoscopy;
6 hirsutism and obesity.

However, halfway through her history the pattern of her menstrual history changes. Whereas she was previously oligomenorrheic, she becomes amenorrheic, and whereas she previously responded to MPA challenge, she is no longer responsive. The lack of response to MPA is usually due to inadequate previous estrogen stimulation of the endometrium, but she was obviously adequately estrogenized. So why did she not have menses following MPA treatment? The reason is that she had developed Asherman's syndrome or uterine scarring following two D&C procedures in the setting of a pregnancy. This was confirmed hysteroscopically and she was treated. Uterine scarring is a potential complication of D&C, especially in the setting of a pregnancy or postpartum. Symptoms include amenorrhea, scanty menses, miscarriages and infertility, and may include significant dysmenorrhea if cervical stenosis is the major component. The adhesions are lysed, usually hysteroscopically, and the patient is treated with high-dose estrogen to promote healing.

Case 124

A 40-year-old patient was referred because of secondary amenorrhea. Her menarche occurred at age 13 years, followed by regular cycles. She took oral contraceptives for a few years and achieved pregnancy at age 29 years, shortly after discontinuing the pill. She had a significant amount of bleeding postpartum, but did not require a transfusion. For a while after this pregnancy she had regular cycles, but by the age of 32 years her menses became less and less regular, and by the age of 34 years she was amenorrheic. Periodic treatment with medroxyprogesterone acetate was always associated with withdrawal bleeding. Her family history was significant for adult-onset diabetes, and she had gained 100 lb (45 kg) in weight over the preceding 10 years. In addition, she complained of scalp hair loss.

Examination
She was overweight at 242 lb (110 kg), and was mildly hirsute, had considerable crown hair thinning and some acanthosis nigricans. There was no galactorrhea, and pelvic examination revealed estrogenic cervical mucus. The uterus was retroverted and no adnexal masses were palpated.

Laboratory Tests
Her prolactin level was 9.0 ng/mL and her thyroid function tests were normal. A suppressed cortisol level of 0.4 μg/dL reflected a therapeutic dexamethasone injection she had received and also ruled out Cushing's syndrome. Her cortisol level subsequently rebounded to 14.2 μg/dL, which is normal. Her testosterone level was 13.6 ng/dL, her DHEA-S was 160 μg/dL, her andostenedione level was 192 ng/dL (normal range 52–200 ng/dL) and her fasting serum insulin was 55.9 μU/mL (normal range 0–20 μU/mL), reflecting her insulin-resistant state. Her glucose and glycosylated hemoglobin levels were normal. Her FSH was unmeasurable, and her LH level was 0.7 IU/L. Her serum estradiol level was 177 pg/mL. A GNRH stimulation of gonadotropin release was performed, and her LH level rose to 3.2 IU/L, but her FSH level remained less than 1 IU/L. MRI of her pituitary revealed a partially empty sella turcica.

Discussion of Case 124

Case 124 presents a diagnostic challenge. She started off with an uneventful reproductive history until after her first and only pregnancy, when she had significant
bleeding, placing her at risk for hypopituitarism (Sheehan's syndrome). However,
fortunately she re-established normal cycles (oligomenorrhea or amenorrhea postpartum almost always occurs in patients with Sheehan's syndrome), but these
became irregular 2 years later and stopped 4 years after her pregnancy. Her amenorrhea was responsive to Provera (medroxyprogesterone acetate) challenge,
indicative of adequate estrogen stimulation of the endometrium. Her amenorrhea,
scalp hair loss, hirsutism and weight gain could have been related to the development of Cushing's syndrome, but a very suppressed cortisol level following a therapeutic dexamethasone injection essentially ruled out this possibility. Her
acanthosis nigricans and increasing obesity together with a strong family history of
diabetes and her very high serum insulin levels in the presence of normal glucose
confirmed her insulin-resistant state. Indeed, her significant male-pattern baldness
was almost certainly related to the excess androgens that are so commonly seen in
insulin-resistant states. However, at the time of her evaluation her serum androgens
levels were normal and her gonadotropins were extremely low, especially given her
age of 40 years. In addition, both LH and especially FSH responded poorly to
GNRH challenge. Even if she had the ovarian hyperandrogenism seen in insulin-
resistant states in the past, her ovarian androgens would *not* be expected to be high
in the presence of such low serum LH levels. The challenge in her case was to
explain her obvious clinical and biochemical evidence of estrogen production
(withdrawal to Provera, mid to late follicular phase serum estradiol, and estrogenic
cervical mucus). Ovarian estradiol production is normally mediated by FSH stimulation, but this patient had unmeasurable FSH, so where was the estradiol coming
from? Her final diagnoses were as follows.

1 Granulosa cell tumor of the ovary producing estradiol and inhibin (her measurably
   elevated inhibin levels were responsible for the suppressed FSH and to a lesser
   extent the LH). The tumor was surgically removed and verified pathologically.
2 Insulin-resistant state with presumed *previous* (i.e. prior to the development of
   her granulosa cell tumor) hyperandrogenism as manifested by her alopecia and
   hirsutism.
3 Partially empty sella, presumed related to her episode of postpartum bleeding,
   but not sufficient to cause clinical or biochemical hypopituitarism.

Case 125

A 50-year-old woman was admitted for management of advanced cervical cancer. At the time of her admission she was very sick. She also had a history of adult-onset diabetes mellitus. On examination, she was found to have severe hirsutism and clitoromegaly. A serum testosterone measurement was obtained and was found to be 20 ng/dL. An endocrine consult was sought to explain the disparity between her physical and laboratory findings.

Examination
The above findings were confirmed. There was no clinical evidence of Cushing's syndrome, and the patient had acanthosis nigricans.

Laboratory Tests
A sample obtained 10 days after the original testosterone measurement showed the following results. The patient was clinically less sick at this time. Her testosterone level was 78 ng/dL, DHEA-S was 54 µg/dL, LH was 2.2 IU/L and FSH was 8.7 IU/L.

Discussion of Case 125

Case 125 could cause great diagnostic confusion if attention is not paid to the chronology of events and time of sampling for hormonal measurements. This patient's acanthosis nigricans, severe hirsutism and clitoromegaly were very suggestive of a severe hyperandrogenic state related to insulin resistance. One would have expected high serum androgens, especially testosterone, but her testosterone level was well within normal limits – hence the dilemma and the need for consultation. Although the ovarian theca/stroma remains active in perimenopausal and menopausal patients and is capable of excess production of androgens, LH stimulation is required for this to occur. In very sick patients, even near-menopausal ones, hypothalamic GNRH production is very significantly impaired, leading to decreased serum gonadotropin levels, especially LH. At the time of this patient's presentation and initial serum testosterone measurement, she was very sick, and although LH was not measured, we can assume that her LH level was very low. Ten days later, she was less sick, her LH was measurable (both her LH and FSH levels were incongruously low for a 50-year-old patient even at this time), and her serum testosterone level was moderately elevated at 78 ng/dL. One can reasonably assume that she had had greater gonadotropin stimulation of her ovarian stroma prior to her illness, given her severe hirsutism and clitoromegaly.

Case 126

A 35-year-old woman was admitted in the 18th week of her pregnancy because of premature rupture of her membranes. An endocrine consult was obtained in order to evaluate severe hirsutism. Her menarche occurred at age 17 years, and she had regular cycles until her first pregnancy at the age of 19 years. A second pregnancy was established at age 21 years. After this pregnancy, her menses became irregular and she developed hirsutism, which increased slowly over the years (including during her current pregnancy). Her voice had also become deeper. In addition, she had gained 110 lb (50 kg) in weight since the age of 17 years. Her mother was diabetic and had some increased hair.

Examination
The patient's voice was husky, and she was moderately to severely hirsute over her face, chin and abdomen. She had acanthosis nigricans and also some clitoromegaly.

Laboratory Tests
Her total testosterone level was 702 ng/dL, her free testosterone level was 5.6 ng/dL (normal range 0.3–1.9 ng/dL) and DHEA-S was 60 μg/dL. Ultrasound examination of her ovaries did not show any evidence of cysts or luteomas.

Case 127

A 24-year-old patient was first evaluated in the middle of her first pregnancy because of a history of deepening of her voice. At this time, her total testosterone level was 411 ng/dL with a free testosterone level of 3.7 ng/dL. By 33 weeks, she had evidence of clitoromegaly. Subsequent delivery by Caesarean section at 38 weeks revealed the presence of 10-cm ovarian luteomas bilaterally. Six weeks postpartum, her total testosterone level was 67 ng/dL, free testosterone was 0.6 ng/dL and DHEA-S was 200 μg/dL. Her total testosterone level was suppressed to 22 ng/dL on a cycle of oral contraceptives. Two years later, she achieved pregnancy again. At 24 weeks' gestation, her total testosterone was 356 ng/dL, and by 29 weeks increased ovarian size was demonstrated bilaterally. By 33 weeks, her total testosterone level was 815 ng/dL, and by 37 weeks it was 1264 ng/dL. At this time she had severe acne and some temporal recession, deepening of her voice (which had improved a little following her last delivery) and definite clitoromegaly. She had a vaginal delivery. Eight weeks postpartum, her total testosterone level was 58 ng/dL.

Discussion of Cases 126 and 127

Case 126 was evaluated because of severe hirsutism in the setting of a pregnancy. In fact, this patient had been hirsute and had deepening of her voice *prior to* her pregnancy. Although she started off with a normal reproductive history, her menses had become irregular after the age of 21 years in association with a very significant weight gain. Her family history of diabetes and her acanthosis nigricans were consistent with an insulin-resistant state, which was presumably aggravated by obesity. Her total serum testosterone level was extremely high, but was partly reflective of a high sex-hormone-binding globulin state characteristic of pregnancy. However, her free testosterone level was also high, consistent with excess androgen production. Ultrasound examination of her ovaries did not reveal any evidence of theca-lutein cysts or luteomas. It is likely that her high serum insulin levels in association with her high HCG concentration (HCG behaves like LH at an ovarian level) combined to stimulate her ovarian stroma, excessively leading to a high androgen state during her pregnancy. Her androgens were also presumed to have been elevated prior to her pregnancy, given her history.

Case 127 developed deepening of her voice and clitoromegaly *during* her first pregnancy, this being associated with very high free testosterone concentrations. Caesarean section revealed bilateral luteomas, which are androgen-producing benign lesions of the ovaries that commonly occur bilaterally and occasionally recur in a subsequent pregnancy, as in this patient. Luteomas are associated with maternal virilization in about one-third of cases. Another cause of excess androgen production in pregnancy is the presence of theca-lutein cysts or hyperreatio luteinalis. These cysts are often associated with conditions resulting in increased human chorionic gonadotropin, such as molar pregnancy and multiple gestation. Maternal virilization occurs in about 30% of cases. Although the hyperandrogenism of theca-lutein cysts is not associated with virilization of a female fetus (thought to relate to placental aromatization of androgens to estrogens), the hyperandrogenism of luteomas may lead to virilization of a female fetus in approximately 80% of the infants born to mothers with virilizing luteomas, and these infants usually exhibit clitoromegaly.

Case 128

A 44-year-old woman attended because of a 4-year history of increasing hirsutism affecting her face, abdomen and chest. She had previously had milder excess hair. Her menarche had occurred at age 12 years, she had her first pregnancy at the age of 18 years, and the second at the age of 23 years. In between, she had taken oral contraceptives. At the age of 28 years, she had a hysterectomy for benign disease. In addition, over time she had gained 100 lb (45 kg) in weight, and in the preceding year she had experienced some hot flashes.

Examination
The patient was moderately hirsute over the affected areas, and she also had a prominent clitoris. There was no clinical evidence of Cushing's syndrome.

Laboratory Tests
Her testosterone level was 197 ng/dL, DHEA-S was 287 μg/dL, LH was 2.9 IU/L and FSH was 4.5 IU/L. Her serum cortisol level was 5.9 μg/dL. Ovarian ultrasound examination revealed normal ovaries measuring 37×25 and 29×28 mm, respectively. Her fasting glucose level was 91 mg/dL and her corresponding insulin level was 21.8 μU/mL (normal range 5–20 μU/mL).

Follow-up
She was treated with a 50-μg estradiol oral contraceptive for one cycle, and a repeat serum testosterone measurement was below the lower limit of detection for that assay.

Discussion of Case 128

Case 128 presented with a 4-year history of increasing hirsutism at the age of 44 years. She had had milder hirsutism previously. She had already been ovulatory, as she had achieved two pregnancies, but she had had no menses after the age of 28 years because of a hysterectomy. Over time, she gained 100 lb (45 kg) in weight, and at the time of her visit she had experienced hot flashes. Laboratory tests revealed an extremely high testosterone level with normal gonadotropins. Cushing's syndrome was essentially ruled out by a baseline cortisol level of 5.9 µg/dL. It was extremely important to rule out an ovarian androgen-producing tumor; her ultrasound examination was normal and her testosterone level was undetectable with gonadotropin suppression. The ovarian stroma remains a viable endocrine organ capable of producing androgens long after follicular exhaustion at menopause, and is increasingly stimulated by rising LH concentrations at this time. This patient's increasing weight was associated with insulin resistance (as evidenced by her high fasting insulin levels). It is likely that her high testosterone levels resulted from the combined effect of LH and insulin stimulation of the ovarian stroma.

Case 129

A 48-year-old patient was seen for management of hormone replacement. After a fairly uneventful reproductive history interrupted by three pregnancies, her menses became erratic at the age of 45 years and she later developed hot flashes. Conjugated equine estrogen (CEE), 0.625 mg, was prescribed together with medroxyprogesterone acetate (MPA), 10 mg for 10 days per month. She was not on this therapy at the time of her initial visit.

Examination
Her blood pressure was 170/90 (repeated later 145/80) mmHg, she was not obese, and physical examination was otherwise unremarkable.

Laboratory Tests
As part of her routine evaluation, thyroid function tests and general chemistry were was obtained. Her thyroid tests were normal, her cholesterol level was 288 mg/dL and her triglyceride level was 240 mg/dL (repeated fasting yielded a level of 213 mg/dL). After replacement with CEE and MPA, her tests were repeated. Her fasting triglyceride level was 3440 mg/dL and cholesterol was 423 mg/dL.

Discussion of Case 129

This patient was mildly hypertriglyceridemic prior to menopausal estrogen replacement therapy. After administration of small doses of conjugated estrogens, her triglyceride levels exceeded 3000 mg/dL, placing her at risk for pancreatitis. She clearly had an underlying lipid disorder which was unmasked by estrogen therapy. It is well known that estrogens affect triglyceride production and occasionally, as in this case, they may unmask a disorder. Transdermal estrogen could have been considered in this case, avoiding first pass through the liver. Raloxifene, which does not elevate triglyceride levels, may also be a suitable alternative.

Glossary of common tests

The hypothalamus produces thyrotropin-releasing hormone (TRH), corti-cotropin-releasing hormone (CRH), gonadotropin-releasing hormone (GNRH), prolactin-inhibiting hormone (dopamine), growth-hormone-releasing hormone (GHRH) and growth-hormone-inhibiting hormone (somatostatin) and other factors. These hormones reach the anterior pituitary via the pituitary portal circulation.

TRH → TSH and prolactin stimulation
GNRH → LH and FSH stimulation
CRH → ACTH stimulation
GHRH → GH stimulation
Dopamine → prolactin inhibition
Somatostatin → GH inhibition

1   The combined test of pituitary function is the gold standard for pituitary hormone reserve. During this test, GNRH (100 μg), TRH (200–500 μg) and insulin (0.1 U/kg) are administered intravenously as boluses, one after the other, after obtaining baseline samples. Blood samples are subsequently obtained every 30 minutes for 2 hours. Peak LH, FSH, prolactin and TSH responses are normally reached at 20–30 minutes. Peak LH > 15 IU/L or a 100% rise is considered normal. An FSH increase of > 50% is also considered normal. TSH increases by at least threefold in normal subjects. A *delayed* rise in TSH is consistent with hypothalamic disease. Prolactin at least doubles in response to TRH, and the response may be greater in females. In excess prolactin states, prolactin concentrations increase further in response to TRH, except in patients with prolactinomas who usually do not respond. Hypoglycemia, which is a potent stimulus for GH and ACTH release, is usually achieved within approximately the first 30 minutes and is followed by release of ACTH (and hence cortisol) and GH. Peak serum cortisol levels exceeding 20 μg/dL and GH exceeding 10 ng/mL in children and 5 ng/mL in adults are considered normal responses. Ovine CRH (1 μg/kg) may also be administered

separately, and a cortisol response exceeding 20 μg/dL within 1 hour is consistent with normal pituitary function.

2 In a clomiphene stimulation test, 100 mg of clomiphene are administered daily for 5 days and the entire hypothalamic–pituitary–gonadal axis is evaluated. LH, FSH and estradiol or testosterone are measured at baseline and on days 6 (day after clomiphene) and 10. Gonadotropin levels should rise by at least 30% (they often double). The levels of steroid sex hormones also rise significantly.

Thyroid

In response to hypothalamic TRH, the pituitary produces TSH, which in turn stimulates the thyroid gland to produce T_4 and T_3, the latter being the active hormone. About 80% of circulating T_3 is actually derived from the peripheral conversion of T_4 to T_3. Both hormones are over 99% bound to proteins such as thyroxine-binding globulin (TBG). Routine thyroid function tests (TFTs) usually consist of total T_4, T_3 resin uptake (T_3RU, a measure of the amount of available binding proteins) and TSH. Using the total T_4 and T_3 resin uptake, a free thyroxine *index* (FTI) can be calculated as follows:

$$T_4 \times T_3RU/100 = FTI$$

Example: $12 \times 33/100 = 4.0$

In states of TBG excess, such as pregnancy or use of oral contraceptives, total T_4 is elevated but conversely T_3RU is suppressed and the FTI is therefore normal.

Example: $15 \times 20/100 = 3.0$

TSH is the most sensitive test of thyroid function, and the availability of second- and third-generation TSH assays allows quantitation of low as well as high levels of TSH. Normal-range TSH reflects euthyroidism; elevated TSH reflects primary hypothyroidism and, except in instances of pituitary/hypothalamic disease, a suppressed TSH is consistent with thyrotoxicosis. Occasionally, in non-thyroidal illness, TSH may be suppressed or elevated in the absence of thyroid disease.

Free T_4 measures the free, bioactive fraction of the total serum T_4. Together with TSH, its measurement is useful when monitoring pregnant patients with thyroid disease. Total T_3 measures predominantly bound hormone, and *free* T_3 measures the free hormone.

Radioactive iodine uptake is measured by administering radioactive iodine, usually ^{123}I, and uptake by the thyroid is recorded at 4–6 and 24 hours. The uptake is elevated in Graves' disease, autonomous nodules and iodine deficiency. It is suppressed in thyroiditis and exogenous thyroid loading. A thyroid scan may also be performed in conjunction with ^{123}I uptake and will image the gland anatomy, showing diffuse or localized uptake.

Antithyroglobulin and antimicrosomal (antithyroid peroxidase) antibodies are both antithyroid antibodies which may be elevated in a variety of autoimmune thyroid diseases, such as Graves' disease, Hashimoto's disease and postpartum thyroiditis. Thyroid-stimulating immunoglobulins (TSI) are TSH-receptor-stimulating antibodies that are found in patients with Graves' disease. They may cross the placenta and cause neonatal thyrotoxicosis.

Adrenal gland

Addison's disease or adrenal insufficiency

Adrenal glucocorticoid reserve is tested for by the administration of 250 µg IV Cortrosyn (synthetic ACTH). Serum cortisol is measured at 30 and 60 minutes. A rise in serum cortisol of > 7 µg/dL from baseline or an absolute cortisol level of ≥ 18 µg/dL during the test is consistent with normal cortisol reserve.

Cushing's syndrome

For the *diagnosis* of Cushing's syndrome, which is a state of cortisol excess, two tests are employed.

Urinary free cortisol

Twenty-four-hour urinary free cortisol (UFC) is measured, and a value of less than 100 µg/24 hours is considered normal. A value greater than twice the upper limit of normal is virtually diagnostic of Cushing's syndrome. False-positive results may be seen in patients with alcoholism or major stress.

Dexamethasone suppression testing

An *overnight* dexamethasone suppression test is a useful *screening* test for Cushing's syndrome. Dexamethasone, 1 mg, is administered at midnight and serum cortisol levels are measured the following morning. A serum cortisol level of < 5 µg/dL rules out Cushing's syndrome.

A *2-day, low-dose* dexamethasone suppression test is a *definitive* test for Cushing's syndrome. Dexamethasone, 0.5 mg, is administered every 6 hours for 8 doses starting at noon of day 1 and ending at 06.00 hours on day 3. A serum cortisol level of < 5 µg/dL on the morning of day 3 rules out Cushing's syndrome.

For the *differential diagnosis* of Cushing's syndrome (adrenal vs. pituitary vs. ectopic ACTH), the following tests are employed.

1   ACTH is measured at 08.00 hours. A value of < 5 pg/mL is consistent with primary adrenal etiology for Cushing's syndrome. ACTH levels of > 500 pg/mL are usually consistent with an ectopic source and value of > 1000 pg/mL are almost always so.

2   A 2-day *high-dose* dexamethasone test is performed by administering 2 mg every 6 hours for 8 doses, starting at 06.00 hours on day 1. Collect 24-hour urine for 17-hydroxycorticosteroids and urinary free cortisol before and during the 2 days of dexamethasone administration. A fall in 17-hydroxycorticosteroids to < 64% of baseline or in 24-hour UFC to < 90% of baseline is consistent with pituitary-dependent Cushing's syndrome (pituitary adenoma).

3   In a CRH stimulation test, ovine CRH, 1 µg/kg body weight, is administered intravenously over 1 minute. Serum cortisol and ACTH levels are measured before and at 15, 30 and 60 minutes after CRH. An increase in ACTH of

$\geq 35\%$ or an increase in cortisol of $\geq 20\%$ from baseline suggests pituitary-dependent Cushing's syndrome. Patients with ectopic ACTH or adrenal tumors fail to augment ACTH or cortisol after CRH. However, ectopic ACTH due to a bronchial carcinoid tumor may respond similarly to pituitary-dependent Cushing's syndrome.

4   A CRH stimulation test with petrosal (or cavernous) sinus sampling, should only be performed by radiologists who are experienced in the use of this procedure. The sinuses are bilaterally cannulated and blood samples obtained both peripherally and from the sinuses before and 2, 5 and 10 minutes after CRH administration. A basal petrosal sinus to periphery (PS/P) ACTH ratio of $> 2:1$ or a post-CRH PS/P ratio of $> 3:1$ identifies the pituitary as the source of ACTH. The test *may* also aid lateralization of the pituitary tumor, although it is not uniformly successful in doing so.

Hirsutism

Obtain a random serum testosterone (preferably follicular phase of cycle) and DHEA-sulfate measurement. Testosterone concentrations of ≥ 200 ng/dL should lead to evaluation for adrenal or ovarian tumors.

An elevated DHEA-S value may be found in the following:

- patients with adrenal hyperandrogenism (most common);
- patients with late-onset congenital adrenal hyperplasia (21-hydroxylase);
- patients with 3-β-hydroxysteroid dehydrogenase deficiency;
- patients with adrenal androgen-producing tumors (DHEA-S > 700 μg/dL).

1   A 2-day low dose (0.5 mg every 6 hours for 8 doses) dexamethasone suppression test will determine the suppressibility of testosterone and DHEA-S. Suppression of testosterone and DHEA-S to $< 50\%$ of baseline values is consistent with adrenal hyperandrogenism. Failure of testosterone to suppress by 50% is consistent with a predominantly ovarian source. Failure to suppress DHEA-S should prompt evaluation for an adrenal tumor that is not responsive to dexamethasone.

2   The ACTH stimulation test is performed for 21-hydroxylase congenital adrenal hyperplasia (CAH) and 3-β-hydroxysteroid dehydrogenase deficiency. Synthetic ACTH (Cortrosyn 250 μg) can be administered intravenously as described above. Blood samples are obtained at baseline, 30 and 60 minutes post-ACTH for 17-OH progesterone and 17-OH pregnenolone. This should be done during the follicular phase of the menstrual cycle.

In CAH 21-hydroxylase deficiency, 17-OH progesterone at baseline is usually > 2 ng/mL and peak levels exceed 10 ng/mL. Partial 3-β-hydroxysteroid dehydrogenase deficiency is suggested by peak 17-OH pregnenolone exceeding 15 ng/mL or a ratio of 17-OH pregnenolone to 17-OH progesterone at 60 minutes of ≥ 8.

Ovary/female reproductive system

1   As described in the section on the hypothalamic–pituitary axis, the clomiphene challenge test evaluates the integrity of the hypothalamic–pituitary–ovarian axis. Clomiphene, acting at the level of the hypothalamus, stimulates GNRH production, which in turn increases the availability of LH and FSH. Increases in LH, FSH and estradiol are consistent with an intact system. An exaggerated FSH response to clomiphene is also consistent with diminished ovarian reserve.

2   With regard to FSH, concentrations of > 30 IU/L are consistent with menopause. Early-cycle (day 3) concentrations exceeding 12 IU/L indicate diminished ovarian reserve.

3   An LH/FSH ratio of > 3 in the follicular phase of the cycle is diagnostic of polycystic ovary syndrome. A ratio of > 2 is highly suggestive of this condition.

4   In a progestin challenge test, medroxyprogesterone acetate, 10 mg, is administered for 5 days. Following withdrawal of this progestin, menstrual bleeding may or may not ensue. The occurrence of bleeding indicates prior stimulation of the endometrium with estrogen *and* an intact outflow tract. The absence of bleeding reflects either the absence of endometrial estrogen stimulation or an outflow tract problem.

5   Outflow tract evaluation may be accomplished in the following ways:
    - progestin challenge as described above;
    - estrogen followed by progestin challenge. Either conjugated estrogen, 1.25 mg, or 17-β-estradiol, 2 mg, may be administered for 25 days. Medroxyprogesterone acetate, 10 mg, is given for the last 10 days of the estrogen therapy. The absence of menstrual flow following this regimen is consistent with an outflow tract problem;
    - a hysterosalpingogram will outline the uterine cavity and can thus demonstrate scarring (Asherman's syndrome), polyps or distortion of the cavity by fibroid tumors. Tubal patency is also shown;
    - hysteroscopy allows direct visualization of the uterine cavity.

Testis/male reproductive system

1   For a semen analysis, see normal laboratory ranges.
2   Perform clomiphene challenge as described above in the section on the hypo-
    thalamic–pituitary axis. It evaluates the integrity of the hypothalamic–
    pituitary–testicular axis. LH, FSH and testosterone concentrations will
    increase following clomiphene challenge.
3   An HCG stimulation test is indicated for the evaluation of Leydig-cell function
    and reserve. An intramuscular injection of 5000 IU of HCG is administered
    and serum testosterone levels are measured before and 3–4 days after the
    injection. An increase in testosterone levels to within the normal range is
    consistent with normal Leydig-cell function.
4   A hamster egg penetration assay evaluates the ability of human sperm to pene-
    trate hamster eggs. A positive test indicates that male fertilizing capacity is
    likely to be normal. A negative result does not always indicate the likelihood of
    lack of fertilization by *in-vitro* fertilization using human eggs, but it suggests that
    there could be a problem.

Laboratory normal ranges

Test	Conventional units	SI units
ACTH	20–100 pg/mL	4–22 pmol/L
Androstenedione: adult female	85–275 ng/dL	3–10 nmol/L
Cholesterol:		
total	≤ 200 mg/dL	< 5.2 mmol/L
HDL	> 35 (M); > 45 (F) mg/dL	> 0.9 (M); > 1.16 (F) mmol/L
LDL	≤ 130 mg/dL	< 3.36 mmol/L
Cortisol:		
a.m.	5–18 µg/dL	140–500 nmol/L
p.m.	2–13 µg/dL	50–360 nmol/L
24-hour urinary free	10–100 µg/day	30–300 nmol/day
DHEA-sulfate: adult female	82–338 µg/dL	2.2–9.2 µmol/L
Estradiol:		
follicular phase	10–100 pg/mL	40–370 pmol/L
mid-cycle	100–230 pg/mL	370–850 pmol/L
luteal phase	10–160 pg/mL	40–590 pmol/L
FSH:		
male:	1–12 IU/L	
female:		
follicular	1–12 IU/L	
postmenopausal	> 30 IU/L	
Glycohemoglobin: non-diabetic	< 6.1%	
Growth hormone	0.0–5.0 ng/mL	< 5 µg/L
Human chorionic gonadotropin:		
non-pregnant	< 5 IU/L	
Insulin (fasting)	5–20 µU/mL	35–145 pmol/L
LH:		
male:	2–12 IU/L	
female:		
follicular	2–12 IU/L	
mid-cycle	18–50 IU/L	
postmenopausal	> 30 IU/L	

Osmolality:
    serum   275–295 mosm/kg
    urine   50–400 mosm/kg

Plasma renin activity   70–330 ng/dL/hour

Progesterone:		
follicular	< 2 ng/mL	< 6 nmol/L
luteal	2–20 ng/mL	6–64 nmol/L
17-OH progesterone: follicular	< 2 ng/mL	< 6 nmol/L
17-OH pregnenolone:	1–3 ng/mL	3–9 nmol/L

Prolactin   2–25 ng/mL   2–25 µg/L

Radioactive ^{123}I uptake:
    4 hours   3–15%
    24 hours   10–35%

Semen analysis:
    volume   1.5–5.0 mL
    count   ≥ 20 million/mL
    motility (1 hour)   ≥ 50%
    morphology (Kruger)   ≥ 14% normal

Testosterone:		
female	≤ 40 ng/dL	< 1.4 nmol/L
male	300–1200 ng/dL	10–42 nmol/L

Thyroid function tests:		
T_4 (total)	4.5–12.5 µg/dL	58–160 nmol/L
T_3 resin uptake	25–35%	0.25–0.35
Free thyroxine index	1.1–4.4	
TSH	0.32–5.00 µIU/mL	0.32–5.00 mU/L
T_3 (total)	60–181 ng/dL	0.92–2.7 nmol/L
T_4 (free)	0.8–1.8 ng/dL	10.3–23 pmol/L

Triglyceride   ≤ 200 mg/dL   < 2.25 nmol/L

References

Cases 1–12

Baird, D.T. 1997: Amenorrhea. *Lancet* **350**, 275.

D'Souza, M.J. 1998: Luteal phase deficiency and anovulation in recreation women runners. *Journal of Clinical Endocrinology and Metabolism* **83**, 4220.

Hayes, F.J., Seminara, S.B. and Crowley, W.F. 1998: Hypogonadotropic hypogonadism. *Endocrinology and Metabolism Clinics of North America* **27**, 739.

McIver, B., Romanski, S.A. and Nippoldt, T.B. 1997: Evaluation and management of amenorrhea. *Mayo Clinic Proceedings* **72**, 1161.

Schwarts, M.W. and Seeley, R.J. 1997: Neuroendocrine responses to starvation and weight loss. *New England Journal of Medicine* **336**, 1802.

Warren, M.P. 1996: Clinical review 77. Evaluation of secondary amenorrhea. *Journal of Clinical Endocrinology and Metabolism* **81**, 437.

Cases 13–26

Conner, P. and Fried, G. 1998: Hyperprolactinemia; etiology, diagnosis and treatment. *Acta Obstetricia et Gynecologica Scandinavica* **77**, 249.

Jeffcoate, W.J., Pound, No, Sturrock, N.D. and Lambourne, J. 1996: Long-term follow-up of patients with hyperprolactinemia. *Clinical Endocrinology* **45**, 299.

Jones, T.H. 1995: The management of hyperprolactinemia. *British Journal of Hospital Medicine* **53**, 374.

Cases 27–33

Bitton, R.N., Slavin, M., Decker, R.E. *et al.* 1991: The course of lymphocytic hypophysitis. *Surgical Neurology* **36**, 40.

Gonzalez-Gonzalez, J.G., Mancillas-Adame, L.G., Lavalle-Gonzalez *et al.* 1997: Transient pituitary enlargement and dysfunction due to lymphocytic hypophysitis. *The Endocrinologist* **7**, 357.

Grimes, H.G. and Brooks, M.H. 1980: Pregnancy in Sheehan's syndrome: report of a case and review. *Obstetrical and Gynecological Survey* **35**, 481.

Meier, C.A. and Biller, M.K.B. 1997: Clinical and biochemical features of Cushing's. *Endocrinology and Metabolism Clinics of North America* **26**, 741.

Nader, S. 1998: Other endocrine disorders of pregnancy. In Creasy, R.K. and Resnick, R. (eds): *Maternal-fetal medicine*, 4th edn. Philadelphia, PA: W.B. Saunders, 1015.

Orth, D.N. 1995: Cushing's syndrome. *New England Journal of Medicine* **332**, 791.

Vance, M.L. 1994: Hypopituitarism. *New England Journal of Medicine* **330**, 1651.

Cases 34–52

Anasti, J.N. 1998: Premature ovarian failure: an update. *Fertility and Sterility* **70**, 1.

Doherty, L., Brown, D.M., Ainslie, M. *et al*: 1997: Turner syndrome practice guidelines. *The Endocrinologist* **7**, 443.

Lippe, B. 1991: Turner syndrome. *Endocrinology and Metabolism Clinics of North America* **20**, 121.

Saenger, P. 1998: Turner's syndrome. *New England Journal of Medicine* **335**, 1749.

Yeung, S.-C.J., Chiu, A.C., Vassilopoulou-Sellin, R. *et al*. 1998: The endocrine effects of nonhormonal antineoplastic therapy. *Endocrine Reviews* **19**, 144.

Case 53

Bloch, M., Schmidt, P.J. and Rubinow, D.R. 1996: Clinical aspects of premenstrual syndrome. *Infertility and Reproductive Medicine Clinics of North America* **7**, 315.

Mezrow, G., Shoupe, D., Spicer, D. *et al*. 1994: Depot leuprolide acetate with estrogen and progestin add-back for longterm treatment of premenstrual syndrome. *Fertility and Sterility* **62**, 932.

Schmidt, P., Neiman, L.K., Danaceau, M.A. *et al*. 1998: Differential behavioral effects of gonadal steroids in women with and in those without premenstrual syndrome. *New England Journal of Medicine* **338**, 209.

Stone, A.B., Pearlstein, T.B. and Brown, W.A. 1990: Fluoxetine in the treatment of premenstrual syndrome. *Psychopharmacology Bulletin* **26**, 331.

Cases 54–72

Azziz, R. and Slayden, S.C. 1996: The 21-hydroxylase-deficient adrenal hyperplasias: more than ACTH hypersecretion. *Journal of the Society for Gynecologic Investigation* **3**, 297.

Ben-Shlomo, I., Homberg, R. and Shalev, E. 1998: Hyperandrogenic anovulation (the polycystic ovary) – back to the ovary? *Human Reproduction Update* **4**, 296.

Dunaif, A. 1995: Hyperandrogenic anovulation (polycystic ovary syndrome): a unique disorder of insulin action associated with an increased risk of non-insulin-dependent diabetes mellitus. *American Journal of Medicine* **98**, 33S.

Ehrmann, D.A., Barnes, R.B. and Rosenfield, R.L. 1995: Polycystic ovary syndrome as a form of functional ovarian hyperandrogenism due to dysregulation of androgen secretion. *Endocrine Reviews* **16**, 322.

Franks, S. 1995: Polycystic ovary syndrome. *New England Journal of Medicine* **333**, 853.

Lajic, S., Wedell, A. The-Hung, B.E. *et al.* 1998: Long-term somatic follow-up of prenatally treated children with congenital adrenal hyperplasia. *Journal of Clinical Endocrinology and Metabolism* **83**, 3872.

Nestler, J.E. 1998: Polycystic ovary syndrome: a disorder for the generalist. *Fertility and Sterility* **70**, 811.

Nestler, J.E., Jakubowicz, D.J., Evans, W.S. *et al.* 1998: Effects of metformin on spontaneous and clomiphene-induced ovulation in the polycystic ovary syndrome. *New England Journal of Medicine* **338**, 1876.

Pang, S. 1998: The molecular and clinical spectrum of 3-beta-hydroxysteroid dehydrogenase deficiency syndrome. *Trends in Endocrinology and Metabolism* **9**, 82.

Rosenfield, R.L. 1996: Evidence that idiopathic functional adrenal hyperandrogenism is caused by dysregulation of adrenal steroidogenesis and that hyperinsulinemia may be involved. *Journal of Clinical Endocrinology and Metabolism* **81**, 878.

Taylor, A.E. 1998: Polycystic ovary syndrome. *Endocrinology and Metabolism Clinics of North America* **27**, 877.

Wild, R.A. 1995: Obesity, lipids, cardiovascular risk and androgen excess. *American Journal of Medicine* **98**, 27S.

Cases 73–80

Brown, R.S. 1996: Autoimmune thyroid disease in pregnant women and their offspring. *Endocrine Practice* **2**, 53.

Freeman, R. 1991: Medical diseases and infertility. *Infertility and Reproductive Medicine Clinics of North America* **2**, 419.

Mestmann, J.H. 1998: Hyperthyroidism in pregnancy. *Endocrinology and Metabolism Clinics of North America* **27**, 127.

Nader, S. and Mastrobattista, J. 1996: Recurrent hyperthyroidism in consecutive pregnancies characterized by hyperemesis. *Thyroid* **6**, 465.

Cases 81–89

Colditz, G.A., Hankinson, S.E., Hunter, D.J. *et al.* 1995: The use of estrogens and progestins and the risk of breast cancer in postmenopausal women. *New England Journal of Medicine* **332**, 1589.

Daly E., Vessey, M.P., Hawkins, M.M. *et al.* 1996: Risk of venous thromboembolism in users of hormone replacement therapy. *Lancet* **348**, 977.

Delmas, P.D., Bjarnason, N.H., Mitlak, B.H. *et al.* 1997: Effects of raloxifene on bone mineral density, serum cholesterol concentrations and uterine endometrium in postmenopausal women. *New England Journal of Medicine* **337**, 1641.

Eastell, R. 1998: Treatment of postmenopausal osteoporosis. *New England Journal of Medicine* **338**, 736.

Johnson, S.R. (ed.) 1997: Menopause and hormone replacement therapy. *Endocrinology and Metabolism Clinics of North America* **26**, 261.

Lindsay, R. 1998: The role of estrogen in the prevention of osteoporosis. *Endocrinology and Metabolism Clinics of North America* **27**, 399.

Locker, G.Y. 1998: Hormonal therapy of breast cancer. *Cancer Treatment Reviews* **24**, 221.

Saag, K.G., Emkey, R., Schnitzer, T.J. *et al.* 1998: Alendronate for the prevention and treatment of glucocorticoid-induced osteoporosis. *New England Journal of Medicine* **339**, 292.

Witt, D.M. and Lousberg, T.R. 1997: Controversies surrounding estrogen use in postmenopausal women. *Annals of Pharmacotherapy* **31**, 741.

Writing Group for the PEPI Trial 1995: Effects of estrogen or estrogen/progestin regimens on heart disease risk factors in postmenopausal women – the Postmenopausal Estrogen/Progestin Interventions (PEPI) Trial. *Journal of the American Medical Association* **273**, 199.

Cases 90–92

Peacock, L.M. and Rock, J.A. 1996: Indication for and technique of myomectomy. *Infertility and Reproductive Medicine Clinics of North America* **7**, 109.

Sullivan, M.W. and Guzick, D.S. 1996: The natural history of uterine myomas. *Infertility and Reproductive Medicine Clinics of North America* **7**, 1.

Cases 93–95

Hurst, B.S. 1992: Treatment options for endometriosis: medical therapies. *Infertility and Reproductive Medicine Clinics of North America* **3**, 645.

Olive, D.L. and Schwartz, L.B. 1993: Endometriosis. *New England Journal of Medicine* **328**, 1759.

Redwine, D.B. 1992: Treatment of endometriosis-associated infertility. *Infertility and Reproductive Medicine Clinics of North America* **3**, 697.

Cases 96–101

Griffin, J.E. 1992: Androgen resistance – the clinical and molecular spectrum. *New England Journal of Medicine* **326**, 611.

Mcwilliams, R.B. and Gibbons, W.E. 1991: Müllerian anomalies and recurrent pregnancy loss. *Infertility and Reproductive Medicine Clinics of North America* **21**, 53.

Cases 102–108

Capri Workshop Group 1998: Male infertility update: the European Society of Human Reproduction and Embryology (ESHRE) Capri Workshop Group. *Human Reproduction* **13**, 2025.

Devroey, P. 1998: Clinical application of new micromanipulative technologies to treat the male. *Human Reproduction* **13** (Suppl. 3), 112.

Forti, G. and Krausz, C. 1998: Evaluation and treatment of the infertile couple. *Journal of Clinical Endocrinology and Metabolism* **83**, 4177.

Hanson, M.A. and Dumeric, D.A. 1998: Initial evaluation and treatment of infertility in a primary-care setting. *Mayo Clinic Proceedings* **73**, 681.

Jones, H.W. and Touer, J.P. 1993: The infertile couple. *New England Journal of Medicine* **329**, 1710.

Cases 109–115

Ansari, A.H. and Kirkpatrick, B. 1998: Recurrent pregnancy loss: an update. *Journal of Reproductive Medicine* **43**, 806.

Carp, H.J.A. Toder, V., Maschiach, S. *et al.* 1990: Recurrent miscarriage: a review of current concepts. *Obstetrical and Gynecological Survey* **45**, 657.

Diamond, M.P. and DeCherney, A.H. (eds) 1996: Recurrent miscarriage. *Infertility and Reproductive Medicine Clinics of North America* **7**, 645.

Case 116

Braunstein, G.D. 1993: Gynecomastia. *New England Journal of Medicine* **328**, 490.

Glass, A.R. 1994: Gynecomastia. *Endocrinology and Metabolism Clinics of North America* **23**, 825.

Cases 117–120

Baker, H.W.G. 1994: Male infertility. *Endocrinology and Metabolism Clinics of North America* **23**, 783.

Handelsman, D.J. 1993: Hypothalamo–pituitary–gonadal axis in chronic renal failure. *Endocrinology and Metabolism Clinics of North America* **22**, 145.

Howard, S.S. 1995: Treatment of male infertility. *New England Journal of Medicine* **332**, 312.

Case 121

Colao, A. and Lombardi, G. 1998: Growth-hormone and prolactin excess. *Lancet* **352**, 1455.

Cases 122–129

DiSaia, P.J., Creasman, W.T., Boronow, R.C. *et al.* 1985: Risk factors and recurrence patterns in Stage I endometrial cancer. *American Journal of Obstetrics and Gynecology* **151**, 1009.

Doyle, M.B. and Lavy, G. 1991: Intrauterine synechiae and pregnancy loss. *Infertility and Reproductive Medicine Clinics of North America* **2**, 91.

Dunaif, A. 1995: Hyperandrogenic anovulation: a unique disorder of insulin action associated with an increased risk of non-insulin-dependent diabetes mellitus. *American Journal of Medicine* **98**, 33S.

Glueck, C.J., Lang, J., Hamer, T. and Tracy, T. 1994: Severe hypertriglyceridemia and pancreatitis when estrogen replacement therapy is given to hypertriglyceridemic women. *Journal of Laboratory and Clinical Medicine*, **123**, 59.

Lappohn, R.E., Burgher, H.G., Bouma, J. *et al.* 1992: Inhibin as a marker for granulosa cell tumor. *Acta Obstetricia et Gynecologica Scandinavica* **71 (Suppl. 155)**, 61.

McClamrock, H.D. and Adashi, E.Y. 1992: Gestational hyperandrogenism. *Fertility and Sterility* **52**, 257.

Van den Berghe, G. de Zegher, F. and Bouillon, R. 1998: Acute and prolonged critical illness as different neuroendocrine paradigms. *Journal of Clinical Endocrinology and Metabolism* **83**, 1827.

Young, R.H. and Scully, R.E. 1992: Endocrine tumors of the ovary. *Current Topics in Pathology* **85**, 114.

Index